T0173781

Carcinoma of an Unknown Primary Site

Carcinoma of an Unknown Primary Site

Edited by

Karim Fizazi
Institut Gustave Roussy
Villejuif, France

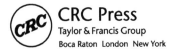

CRC Press
Taylor & Francis Group
Boca Raton London New York

CRC Press is an imprint of the
Taylor & Francis Group, an **informa** business

A TAYLOR & FRANCIS BOOK

First published 2006 by Taylor & Francis

Published 2019 by CRC Press
Taylor & Francis Group
6000 Broken Sound Parkway NW, Suite 300
Boca Raton, FL 33487-2742

© 2006 by Taylor & Francis Group, LLC
CRC Press is an imprint of Taylor & Francis Group, an Informa business

First issued in paperback 2019

No claim to original U.S. Government works

ISBN 13: 978-0-367-45369-5 (pbk)
ISBN 13: 978-0-8247-2799-4 (hbk)

This book contains information obtained from authentic and highly regarded sources. Reasonable efforts have been made to publish reliable data and information, but the author and publisher cannot assume responsibility for the validity of all materials or the consequences of their use. The authors and publishers have attempted to trace the copyright holders of all material reproduced in this publication and apologize to copyright holders if permission to publish in this form has not been obtained. If any copyright material has not been acknowledged please write and let us know so we may rectify in any future reprint.

Except as permitted under U.S. Copyright Law, no part of this book may be reprinted, reproduced, transmitted, or utilized in any form by any electronic, mechanical, or other means, now known or hereafter invented, including photocopying, microfilming, and recording, or in any information storage or retrieval system, without written permission from the publishers.

For permission to photocopy or use material electronically from this work, please access www.copyright.com (http://www.copyright.com/) or contact the Copyright Clearance Center, Inc. (CCC), 222 Rosewood Drive, Danvers, MA 01923, 978-750-8400. CCC is a not-for-profit organization that provides licenses and registration for a variety of users. For organizations that have been granted a photocopy license by the CCC, a separate system of payment has been arranged.

Trademark Notice: Product or corporate names may be trademarks or registered trademarks, and are used only for identification and explanation without intent to infringe.

Visit the Taylor & Francis Web site at
http://www.taylorandfrancis.com

and the CRC Press Web site at
http://www.crcpress.com

Library of Congress Cataloging-in-Publication Data

Carcinoma of an unknown primary site / edited by Karim Fizazi.
     p. ; cm.
  Includes bibliographical references and index.
  ISBN-13: 978-0-8247-2799-4 (alk. paper)
  ISBN-10: 0-8247-2799-1 (alk. paper)
  1. Cancer of unknown primary origin. I. Fizazi, Karim.
  [DNLM: 1. Neoplasms, Unknown Primary--diagnosis--Case reports. 2.
Carcinoma--diagnosis--Case Reports. 3. Carcinoma--therapy--Case Reports. 4. Neoplasms, Unknown
Primary--therapy--Case Reports. QZ 202 C2897 2006]

RC268.48.C39 2006
616.99'4--dc22
                                      2005046647

Library of Congress Card Number 2005046647

Preface

Talking about the unknown is not a typical task for scientists; it is a subject usually more familiar to erudite religious persons. This is one of the reasons why writing and editing a book on carcinomas of an unknown primary site was a challenge. These neoplasms are characterized by a specific and unique phenotype: early and usually aggressive metastatic dissemination with no identifiable primary tumor. When faced with a patient presenting such malignanices, the questions the oncologist must typically address are as follows: "Should I search for the primary or not?" "If so, how should I proceed: use conventional radiology? endoscopies? PET scan?" "Could immunohistochemistry or even genomics be contributive?" As the primary tumor is not usually found, the next series of questions may typically be: "Is it a specific carcinoma of an unknown primary site entity requiring a particular treatment?" "If not, should I use a regimen with a wide anticancer spectrum of activity?" "Is there evidence for a better regimen in terms of progression-free survival or overall survival" "How can I assess the prognosis in this individual case?" "Is there an ongoing clinical trial worth considering for this patient with a carcinoma of an unknown primary site?"

To try to answer these questions, I was delighted to receive favorable and often enthusiastic replies from a number of oncologists and nononcologists in six countries from Europe and America whom I contacted to co-author this book, which to my knowledge is the first of its kind. In order to give the reader the most objective information and the most balanced appraisal on the subject, our policy was to have chapters written by at least two contributors from different groups and countries when applicable.

Finally, it seemed to us didactic and useful to the reader to illustrate the information contained in the chapters by providing a series of comprehensive clinical cases, some of which describe typical carcinoma of unknown primary site cases, while others describe exceptional and challenging settings. Once again, the policy was to have these clinical cases written by an expert in carcinomas of an unknown primary site, with another contributor from a different country making a comment and putting the case into perspective.

Looking at the final result, I feel that it has more than fulfilled my initial hopes and expectations, and that the tremendous efforts required to get such a book written were definitely worth it. This is why I would like to thank all of the contributors and Taylor & Francis Health Sciences for having made this book a reality. Most of all, we collectively hope that this book will contribute to a better outcome for patients with carcinoma of an unknown primary site, thanks to better clinical care and improved clinical and translational research.

Karim Fizazi

Contents

Preface . . . . *iii*

Contributors . . . . *xiii*

SECTION I: CARCINOMAS OF UNKNOWN PRIMARY SITE: SEVERAL THINGS WE KNOW FOR SURE

1. **What We Know About Carcinomas of Unknown Primary Site (CUP) *Almost* for Sure: Incidence, Survival, and Necropsy Data** *1*
   Agnès J. Van de Wouw and Agnès Laplanche
   Introduction 2
   Incidence and Mortality 2
   Clinical Behavior of CUP 5
   Autopsy Data 6
   Survival 7
   References 8

SECTION II: DIAGNOSTIC EVALUATION IN CARCINOMAS OF UNKNOWN PRIMARY SITE: WHAT SHALL WE DO AND WHEN SHALL WE STOP SEEKING THE PRIMARY SITE?

2. **Radiographic Studies, Endoscopy, and Serum Tumor Markers in the Diagnostic Evaluation of Carcinomas of Unknown Primary Site** *11*
   Gauri R. Varadhachary and Renato Lenzi
   Introduction 11

Chest X Ray 13

Computed Axial Tomography 14

Contrast Studies of the GI Tract and Endoscopic
Procedures 16

Serum Tumor Markers 18

Survival Patterns and Their Effect on Diagnostic Strategies in
Patients Presenting with Occult Primary Cancer 19

Conclusion and Future Directions 21

References 22

**3. The Advent of Immunohistochemistry in Carcinoma of Unknown
Primary Site: A Major Progress** *25*
*Jean-Jacques Voigt, Marie-Christine Mathieu, and
Frédéric Bibeau*

Introduction 25

Methods 26

Strategies for Specific Histopathological Types 30

Strategies Depending on Anatomic Localization 32

Targeted Treatment of CUP 32

Conclusion 33

References 33

4. The Importance of Identifying CUP Subsets *37*
Nicholas Pavlidis and Yacine Merrouche

Introduction 37

Histopathological Subtypes 38

Clinicopathological Entities 39

Favorable Subsets 40

Unfavorable Subsets 43

References 45

SECTION III: EMERGING DIAGNOSTIC TOOLS

**5. Role of Positron Emission Tomography with
18F-Fluorodesoxyglucose (PET-FDG) in the Care of
Carcinomas of an Unknown Primary Site** *49*
Etienne Garin and Dirk Rades

Introduction 49

PET-FDG and Cervical Metastases of Unknown
Primary 51

PET-FDG and CUP Not Targeted on Cervical
    Metastases 55
Conclusions 57
References 58

SECTION IV: PROGNOSTIC FACTORS

**6. Prognostic Considerations in Patients with Unknown
Primary Carcinoma** *61*
Renato Lenzi and Stéphane Culine
Introduction 61
Prognostic Factors in UPC Patients with PDC
    and PDA 63
Prognostic Factors in the General Population of
    UPC Patients 68
Prognostic Factors and UPC Clinical Trials 73
Conclusion 74
References 75

SECTION V: SYSTEMIC CHEMOTHERAPY

**7. Treatment of Patients with Favorable Subsets of
Unknown Primary Carcinoma** *79*
John D. Hainsworth
Introduction 79
Women with Peritoneal Carcinomatosis 79
Women with Axillary Lymph Node Metastases 81
Adenocarcinoma Presenting as a Single Metastatic
    Lesion 81
Young Men with Features of Extragonadal Germ Cell
    Tumor 82
Squamous Carcinoma Involving Cervical
    Lymph Nodes 82
Squamous Carcinoma Involving Inguinal
    Lymph Nodes 83
Neuroendocrine Carcinoma with an Unknown
    Primary Site 84
Poorly Differentiated Carcinoma 86

Conclusion 88
References 88

8. **Chemotherapy for Patients with Metastatic Carcinoma of
   Unknown Primary Site** *93*
   F. Anthony Greco and Stéphane Culine
   Introduction 93
   Historical Background 94
   The Minnie Pearl Cancer Research Network
      Experience 95
   The French Experience 95
   At the End, Does Chemotherapy Improve
      Survival? 98
   Conclusion 101
   References 101

9. **Randomized Trials in Patients with Carcinoma
   of an Unknown Primary Site: The Past, the Present,
   and the Future** *105*
   Karim Fizazi and Hans-Joachim Schmoll
   Introduction 105
   Methods 106
   Results 110
   References 114

**SECTION VI: LOCAL TREATMENTS IN CARCINOMA OF
UNKNOWN PRIMARY SITE: IS IT RELEVANT?**

10. **Squamous Cell Carcinoma of an Unknown Primary Tumor
    Located in the Cervical Lymph Nodes** *117*
    Marie-Christine Kaminsky and Emmanuel Blot
    Summary 117
    Introduction 118
    Epidemiology 118
    Patient Work-Up 118
    The Role of PET 119
    Staging 120
    Prognosis 120
    Treatment 121
    Follow-Up 122
    References 123

11. **Women with Isolated Adenocarcinoma in the Axillary Lymph Node of an Unknown Primary Site** *127*
   A. Lortholary, C. El Kouri, J. F. Ramée, and P. Kerbrat
   Introduction 127
   Incidence 128
   Presentation 128
   Para-Clinical Examinations 128
   Treatment 129
   Prognosis 130
   Conclusion 130
   References 130

12. **Carcinoma of Unknown Primary in a Single Site** *133*
   Thierry Lesimple and Carmen Balaña
   Introduction 133
   Differential Diagnosis and Paraclinic
      Investigations 134
   Localized Lymph-Node Metastases of a CUP 135
   Liver Metastasis from a CUP in a Single Site 137
   Isolated Bone Metastasis 138
   Solitary Pulmonary Nodule from a CUP 139
   Localized Pleural Effusion of a CUP 140
   Single Cerebral Metastasis of a CUP 141
   Metastasis of Cutaneous or Soft Tissues from
      a CUP 143
   Conclusion 143
   References 143

13. **Emerging Local Treatments in Carcinomas of an Unknown Primary Site: Radiofrequency, Palliative Bone Surgery, and Radiotherapy** *147*
   D. Pasquier, E. Lartigau, F. Bonodeau, G. Missenard, C. Court, and B. Meunier
   Introduction 147
   Radiofrequency 148
   Palliative Bone Surgery 149
   Radiotherapy 153
   References 155

SECTION VII: THE BIOLOGY OF CARCINOMA OF UNKNOWN PRIMARY SITE

14. The Biology of Unknown Primary Tumors: The Little We Know, the Importance of Learning More *159*
Pierre Busson, Leela Daya-Grosjean, Nicholas Pavlidis, and Agnès J. Van de Wouw
Introduction 159
Nosological Considerations 160
Research Aims and Instruments 161
Brief Summary of Current Knowledge on the Metastatic
    Phenotype 163
Specific and Nonspecific Biological Features
    of UPTs 164
What Is the p53 Status in UPTs? 165
Acquisition of the Metastatic Phenotype in UPTs: From
    Speculation to Testable Hypotheses 166
The Enigma of Primary Tumor Growth Inhibition 167
Search for Prognostic Biological Indicators and Assessment of
    Potential Molecular Targets 169
Conclusion 171
References 171

SECTION VIII: QUALITY OF LIFE AND PSYCHOSOCIAL ASPECTS

15. Psychosocial Aspects of Cancer of Unknown Primary Site *175*
Renato Lenzi, Walter F. Baile, Chantal Rodary, and Patricia A. Parker
Introduction 175
Psychosocial Adjustment and Cancer 177
Assessment and Prevalence of Psychosocial Distress in
    Patients with Known Primary Cancers and in Patients
    with CUP 178
Aspects of Psychosocial Adjustment in CUP Patients: Illness
    Uncertainty, Depression, Anxiety, and Perception of
    Physician's Supportive Behavior 179
QOL Instruments in CUP 181

Diagnosis, Prognosis, and Treatment Plan: Preliminary
  Findings in CUP Patients 182
Challenging Physician–Patient Communication
  Tasks in CUP 183
Conclusion 189
References 190

SECTION IX: CLINICAL CASES OF CARCINOMA OF UNKNOWN PRIMARY SITE

**Case 1: A Female Patient with Pleural Extension of an Unknown
  Primary Carcinoma** *Karim Fizazi* 195
  Comment *F. Anthony Greco* 196

**Case 2: A Favorable Case of CUP with Peritoneal
  Adenocarcinomatosis** *Nicholas Pavlidis* 199
  Comment *Thierry Lesimple* 200

**Case 3: Clear Cell Adenocarcinoma Presenting as a Carcinoma
  of Unknown Primary Origin** *Carmen Balaña,
  Eva Castellà, and Rafael Rosell* 201

**Case 4: A Female Patient with a Single-Site Carcinoma
  of an Unknown Primary Located on the
  Thoracic Wall** *Karim Fizazi and Sylvie Bonvalot* 208
  Comment *Nicholas Pavlidis* 209

**Case 5: An Unfavorable Case of CUP with Metastatic
  Adenocarcinoma to the Liver and Bones**
  Nicholas Pavlidis 211
  Comment *Yacine Merrouche* 212

**Case 6: A Favorable Case of CUP with Metastatic Adenocarcinoma
  of the Liver with Neuroendocrine Differentiation**
  Nicholas Pavlidis 214
  Comment *Stéphane Culine* 215

Case 7: Carcinoma or Melanoma of an Unknown Primary?
  Emmanuel Blot and Sophie Laberge-Le-Couteulx 216
  Comment *Yacine Merrouche* 217

Case 8: A Male Patient with HIV Infection and Carcinoma of an Unknown Primary Site *Roland Bugat* 218
Comment *A. Plantade, P. Afchain, and C. Louvet* 220

Case 9: A 66-Year-Old Male with Liver Metastases of an Unknown Primary Site *Roland Bugat* 223
Comment *A. Plantade, P. Afchain, and C. Louvet* 224

Case 10: An Undifferentiated Carcinoma of an Unknown Primary of the Middle Line in a Young Adult *Roland Bugat* 227
Comment *A. Plantade, P. Afchain, and C. Louvet* 229

Case 11: A Female with Bone Metastases of an Unknown Primary Site *Roland Bugat* 231
Comment *A. Plantade, P. Afchain, and C. Louvet* 233

Index *237*

Contributors

P. Afchain Hôpital Saint Antoine, Paris, France

Walter F. Baile Department of Neuro–Oncology, Section of Psychiatry, The University of Texas M.D. Anderson Cancer Center, Houston, Texas, U.S.A.

Carmen Balaña Medical Oncology Service and Pathology Department, Institut Catalá D'Oncologia, Hospital Germans Trias i Pujol, Barcelona, Spain

Frédéric Bibeau Department of Pathology, Centre Val d'Aurelle, Montpellier, France

Emmanuel Blot Centre Henri Becquerel, Rouen, France

F. Bonodeau Department of Radiology, Centre O. Lambret, Lille, France

Sylvie Bonvalot Institut Gustave Roussy, Villejuif, France

Roland Bugat Institut National du Cancer (INCa), Paris, France

Pierre Busson CNRS UMR 8126, Institut Gustave Roussy, Villejuif, France

Eva Castellà Medical Oncology Service, Institut Catalá D'Oncologia, Hospital Germans Trias i Pujol, Barcelona, Spain

C. Court Department of Orthopaedic Surgery, Kremlin Bicêtre Hospital, Paris Sud University, Paris, Leclerc, France

Stéphane Culine Centre Val d'Aurelle, Montpellier, France

Leela Daya-Grosjean CNRS UPR 2169, Institut Gustave Roussy, Villejuif, France

C. El Kouri Centre Catherine de Sienne, Nantes, France

Karim Fizazi Institut Gustave Roussy, Villejuif, France

Etienne Garin Nuclear Medicine Department, Eugene Marquis Centre, Rennes, France

F. Anthony Greco Sarah Cannon Research Institute, Nashville, Tennessee, U.S.A.

John D. Hainsworth Sarah Cannon Research Institute, Nashville, Tennessee, U.S.A.

Marie-Christine Kaminsky Department of Medical Oncology, Centre Alexis Vautrin, Vandoeuvre Les-Nancy, France

P. Kerbrat Centre Eugène Marquis, Rennes, France

Sophie Laberge-Le-Couteulx Centre Henri Becquerel, Rouen, France

Agnès Laplanche Department of Biostatistics and Epidemiology, Institut Gustave Roussy, Villejuif, France

E. Lartigau Department of Radiation Oncology, Centre O. Lambret, University Lille II, Lille, France

Renato Lenzi Department of Gastrointestinal Medical Oncology, The University of Texas M.D. Anderson Cancer Center, Houston, Texas, U.S.A.

Thierry Lesimple Clinical Research Unit, Comprehensive Cancer Centre Eugène Marquis, Rennes, France

A. Lortholary Centre Catherine de Sienne, Nantes, France

C. Louvet Hôpital Saint Antoine, Paris, France

Marie-Christine Mathieu Department of Pathology, Institut Gustave Roussy, Villejuif, France

Yacine Merrouche Institut de Cancérologie de la Loire, Saint Priest en Jarez, France

B. Meunier Department of Oncological Surgery, Pontchaillou Hospital, Rennes, France

G. Missenard Department of Surgery, Clinique Arago, Paris, France

Patricia A. Parker Department of Behavioral Science, The University of Texas M.D. Anderson Cancer Center, Houston, Texas, U.S.A.

D. Pasquier Department of Radiation Oncology, Centre O. Lambret, University Lille II, Lille, France

Nicholas Pavlidis Department of Medical Oncology, Ioannina University Hospital, Ioannina, Greece

A. Plantade Hôpital Saint Antoine, Paris, France

Dirk Rades Department of Radiation Oncology, University Medical Center Hamburg–Eppendorf, Hamburg, Germany

J. F. Ramée Centre Catherine de Sienne, Nantes, France

Chantal Rodary Department of Public Health, Institut Gustave Roussy, Villejuif, France

Rafael Rosell Medical Oncology Service, Institut Catalá D'Oncologia, Hospital Germans Trias i Pujol, Barcelona, Spain

Hans-Joachim Schmoll Martin-Luther University, Halle, Germany

Agnès J. Van de Wouw Department of Internal Medicine, Slingeland Hospital Doetinchem, The Netherlands

Gauri R. Varadhachary Department of Gastrointestinal Medical Oncology, The University of Texas M.D. Anderson Cancer Center, Houston, Texas, U.S.A.

Jean-Jacques Voigt Department of Pathology, Institut Claudius Regaud, Toulouse, France

——————— **1** ———————

What We Know About Carcinomas of Unknown Primary Site (CUP) *Almost* for Sure: Incidence, Survival, and Necropsy Data

Agnès J. Van de Wouw

Department of Internal Medicine, Slingeland Hospital Doetinchem, The Netherlands

Agnès Laplanche

Department of Biostatistics and Epidemiology, Institut Gustave Roussy, Villejuif, France

There is a wide variation in carcinoma of unknown primary site (CUP) mortality and incidence rates across countries reported in publications, which may mainly be explained by:

1. *Variations in definition.* In many countries, CUP is not identified separately and the diagnosis is not always histologically proven.
2. *The population described.* Epidemiological data concerning CUP are rarely provided by cancer registries and most of the research data on CUP come from tertiary referral centers.

CUP represents 2% to 4% of all cancers among males and females and is slightly more frequent among males. The median age at presentation is approximately 65 to 70 years; CUP is extremely rare in children. Survival is poor, with a median equal to 11 weeks and a one-year survival rate of 15%.

Box 1
Pathological Classification of CUP

- Adenocarcinoma
- Squamous Cell Carcinoma
- Poorly Differentiated Carcinoma
- Undifferentiated Neoplasm

INTRODUCTION

CUP is an intriguing clinical finding that is defined as biopsy-proven metastasis from a malignancy in the absence of an identifiable primary site after a complete history and physical examination, basic laboratory studies, chest X ray, and additional directed studies indicated by positive findings during the initial work-up (1). How long the primary is unknown is not mentioned in this definition. Proposals have been made to integrate a "time factor" into the definition of CUP, but to date, no definite time factor has been used, mainly because thorough analysis of the patient and pathological material takes time (2,3).

A careful and comprehensive pathological examination of biopsied metastatic lesions is crucial for the diagnosis of CUP (see Chapter 4). These tumors can be divided into the following pathological groups: adenocarcinoma (50–70%), squamous cell carcinoma (5–8%), poorly differentiated carcinoma (20–30%), and undifferentiated neoplasm (2–3%) (Box 1) (4–10). Neuroendocrine carcinoma (2–4%) is often mentioned separately because this entity belongs to a treatable subgroup as it is often equated with small cell lung carcinoma and treated as such. Immunohistochemical staining and monoclonal antibodies can be helpful in identifying the nature of tumors. Regretfully, the specificity for the most common markers, which can help unearth the primary site, is not conclusive (11,12).

A big mystery is the underlying biology of this tumor. Scientists are still debating whether CUP is a biological entity or simply metastases shed by a well-hidden primary. Further on in this book, the specific clinical and pathological diagnostic tools, treatment, and biological behavior are discussed.

INCIDENCE AND MORTALITY

There is a wide variation in CUP figures reported in publications (0.5–10%), which may mainly be explained by variations in: (1) definition, (2) time period, and (3) population described (6–8,13–16).

> *Definition*: In many countries CUP is not identified separately, although the 9th edition of International Classification of Diseases for Oncology (ICD-O) provided codes 196-199 referring to different

sites of metastatic malignancy of unknown primary and code C80.9 has been provided specifically for CUP in the 10th edition of the ICD-O. The incidence of CUP can be under- as well as overestimated by changing the definition. Overestimation can occur when the diagnosis is not microscopically confirmed, in which case, patients with benign disease or lymphoma can then be included. The diagnosis is not histologically confirmed in 20% to 25% of the patients (6,7,13). This is a major problem because the diagnosis should be histologically proved, but this practice is so common that this large group of patients cannot be ignored. Lack of histological confirmation can also lead to underestimation: in many countries, CUP is diagnosed only at autopsy, so these patients are not included. Underestimation can also occur when primary sites are "assigned" to patients on a best-guess basis in the absence of positive proof (13,17).

Time Period: The lack of histologically proven diagnoses is currently on the decrease because patients have greater access to medical care, so they are in a better clinical condition when diagnosed. Microscopic confirmation occurs more frequently, thereby excluding other diagnoses and additional directed studies, indicated more often as a result of positive findings during the initial work-up, and reveals more primaries. Furthermore, new sophisticated diagnostic techniques such as the PET scan and microarray technologies, currently available, also identify the primary in a certain percentage of patients.

Described Population: Epidemiological data concerning CUP are rarely provided by cancer registries and most of the research data on CUP come from tertiary referral centers. In order to be valid, epidemiological data must be population-based, consequently only cancer registry figures obtained by interrogating the European Network of Cancer Registries (EUROCIM) database (18) are reported.

Table 1 presents by sex, the mortality rates (per 100,000) observed in 1997 in 16 European countries (18). CUP is coded 196-199 using ICD-O-9 and all rates are standardized on the world population. CUP mortality rates are slightly more elevated among males than among females, but the most striking fact is the wide range in CUP mortality rates across countries (3×10^{-5} in Austria to 14×10^{-5} in the United Kingdom among males), which can be explained by death certification practices at local level. Table 2 presents by sex, CUP (ICD-O-10: C80.9) incidence rates (per 100,000 and standardized on the world population) observed in 1997 in the European registries covering a population exceeding 3 million persons (18). The wide variation observed across countries for mortality is also observed for incidence data, although they were recorded with the specific ICD-O-10 code for CUP. It is noteworthy that this variation can be observed in the

Table 1 1997 Age Standardized (World) Mortality Rates (per 100,000)

Country	Male	Female
Austria	3.2	2.3
Finland	3.9	2.8
Iceland	4.0	4.0
Sweden	4.1	3.7
Italy	4.7	2.4
Portugal	6.3	3.1
Germany	7.1	4.5
Greece	7.6	5.4
Switzerland	7.7	4.8
Norway	7.9	5.7
Ireland	9.3	6.8
France	9.6	5.0
Denmark	9.7	7.9
Netherlands	10.0	6.5
Spain	10.2	4.9
United Kingdom	14.2	10.3

Source: From ICD-O-9: 196-199.

Table 2 1997 Age Standardized (World) Incidence Rates (per 100,000)

Registry[a]	Male	Female
Belgium (Flanders)	5.4	4.5
Croatia	3.7	1.8
Czech-republic	2.5	1.6
Finland	3.3	3.0
Ireland	7.3	6.7
Lithuania	1.0	0.7
Netherlands	10.4	6.8
Norway	4.8	5.0
Russia (St. Petersburg)	2.5	1.4
Slovakia	0.6	0.2
United Kingdom (northwest)	2.4	2.5
United Kingdom (south; Thames)	11.7	9.2
United Kingdom (Scotland)	9.0	7.8
United Kingdom (southwest)	3.6	3.2
United Kingdom (Trent)	11.6	8.9
United Kingdom (Yorkshire)	15.3	10.3

[a]European registries with population >3 million.
Source: From ICD-O-10: C80.9.

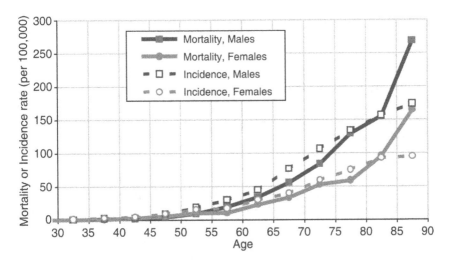

Figure 1 Mortality and incidence rates (ICD-O-9: 196-199) in The Netherlands in 1997. *Abbreviation*: ICD-O, International Classification of Diseases for Oncology.

same country (United Kingdom) across registries. CUP is slightly more frequent among males than among females and represents 2% to 4% of all cancers among males and females (6,15,19,20).

In the Netherlands, CUP represents about 4% of all new cancers and is ranked the seventh most common cancer in males and the eighth in females, which means that it is more common than non-Hodgkin's lymphoma. Cancer Registry data over the 1989 to 2000 period showed that the CUP incidence rate remained unchanged. The fact that a biopsy was performed in a greater percentage of the patients had no influence on the incidence rate.

The median age at presentation is approximately 65 to 70 years (6,15,19), and CUP is extremely rare among children (6,15,19). Figure 1 presents the incidence and mortality rates by age observed in 1997 in the Netherlands (ICD-O-9: 196-199) (21). Survival is poor, with a median equal to 11 weeks (6) and a one-year survival rate of 15% (6,15).

CLINICAL BEHAVIOR OF CUP

Although CUP is a heterogeneous group of tumors with widely diverse natural histories, clinically, they exhibit common typical characteristics (Box 2) (21,22).

First, patients predominantly present with a short history of non-specific complaints (anorexia, weight loss, etc.) (24). Second, the primary tumor remains in most cases unidentified throughout life. Exact figures concerning this issue are missing because different search methods are used

Box 2
Clinical Behavior of CUP

- Short History of Nonspecific Complaints
- Primary Remains Unidentified in Most Cases
- 30% Present with over Three Metastatic Sites
- Unusual Pattern of Distant Spread
- Poor Prognosis

(intensive search, clinical follow-up), most data are collected retrospectively, and different CUP populations are used. In two studies, the primary tumor site was identified antemortem in 11% to 20% of the patients by an extensive radiographic and/or endoscopic search (23,25). Hainsworth et al. studied only patients with neuroendocrine carcinoma and found the primary in 4/29 patients (26). In three other retrospective studies the primary was revealed during the clinical follow-up after the diagnosis in 5% to 15% of the patients (27–29).

Third, approximately 30% of patients with CUP present with three or more organs involved (6,8,9,27,30,31). This differs considerably from the percentage of patients with three or more involved organs in metastasised known primaries, which is below 15% (32–34). Fourth, an unusual pattern of distant spread has been reported in some large autopsy studies (10,25,35). Differences in metastatic sites were observed, when the primary tumor was found at autopsy and the pattern of spread of CUP was compared with the common sites of distant dissemination from known primary tumors (see Autopsy Data). Fifth, patients with CUP have a very poor prognosis, if treatable subgroups are excluded.

AUTOPSY DATA

A postmortem examination is performed in only a minority of patients with CUP (14,23,25,27–29,36,37). Even after thorough evaluation at autopsy, only 55% to 85% of the primaries are found in patients with CUP and when found, they are usually small asymptomatic tumors (10,14,25,35,37). The primary tumor is mainly found in the pancreas (20–26%) and lung (17–23%). Other primary sites are the colon or rectum (4–10%), liver (3–11%), stomach (3–8%), kidney (4–6%), ovary (3–4%), prostate (3–4%), breast (2%), and other (< 2%). A relatively high number of metastases in CUP are found in the kidney, adrenal gland, skin, and heart, when compared with expected sites of metastasis (32).

Selection bias is of obvious concern in any study based on autopsy data. In two retrospective studies, patient characteristics and tumor-specific parameters of autopsied and non-autopsied patients were compared and did not differ from each other, making a significant selection bias unlikely (14,27).

SURVIVAL

In registry populations, patients with CUP have a poor prognosis with a median survival of three to five months and a one-year survival rate of less than 20% (6,7,10,15,23,38). From the older studies it became obvious that some patients responded better to specific treatment than others, and treatable subgroups with a better prognosis due to specific treatment were recognized (Box 3). These groups and therapies will be dealt with in detail in Chapters 4 and 7.

In some recent studies with selected patients from poor prognostic groups, median survival from 6 to 13 months was attained with 25% to 40% of patients alive one year after the diagnosis (8,9,39–49). These data cannot be generalized because they were mainly collected in phase II studies performed in secondary and tertiary referral centers. On the other hand, patients belonging to recognized treatable subgroups were typically excluded from these studies. Caution should therefore be exercised before extrapolating these figures to all CUP patients. When patient characteristics in unselected populations were compared to those of long-term survivors, patients who experienced a lower rate of survival were older; the diagnosis was more often made clinically and they received less treatment (6). Patients are therefore selected before further diagnostic work-up and treatment. Patients who are more likely to benefit from therapy can be selected by using prognostic models developed by van der Gaast and Culine (31,50). The most important prognostic factors are the performance status, serum lactate dehydrogenase, and serum alkaline phosphatase (see Chapter 6). With

Box 3
Treatable Subgroups

- Patients with Squamous Cell Carcinoma (SCC) Involving the Upper or Mid-cervical Lymph Nodes
- Patients with SCC Involving the Inguinal Lymph Nodes
- Female Patients with Axillary Lymph Node Metastases
- Women with Peritoneal Carcinomatosis
- Men with Skeletal Metastases and/or Increased Prostate Specific Antigen
- Poorly Differentiated Adenocarcinoma and Poorly Differentiated Carcinoma
- Poorly Differentiated Neuroendocrine Tumors
- Resectable Metastasis

recent techniques such as microarray technology, more accurate prognostic profiles are likely to be identified, so better patient selection can be achieved before deciding which type of treatment to propose (chemotherapy or other antitumor therapies).

REFERENCES

1. Abbruzzese JL, Abbruzzese MC, Lenzi R, Hess KR, Raber MN. Analysis of a diagnostic strategy for patients with suspected tumors of unknown origin. J Clin Oncol 1995; 13(8):2094–2103.
2. Abbruzzese JL, Abbruzzese MC, Lenzi R, Raber MN, Hess KR. Are time or intensity factors important to the definition of metastases of unknown origin? J Natl Cancer Inst 1996; 88(7):462–463.
3. Barista I, Celik I, Gullu I, Hayran M, Akova M. Integrating the time factor into the definition of metastasis of unknown origin. J Natl Cancer Inst 1996; 88(1):51.
4. Lembersky BC, Thomas LC. Metastases of unknown primary site. Med Clin North Am 1996; 80(1):153–171.
5. Daugaard G. Unknown primary tumors. Cancer Treat Rev 1994; 20(2):119–147.
6. van de Wouw AJ, Janssen-Heijnen ML, Coebergh JW, Hillen HF. Epidemiology of unknown primary tumors; incidence and population-based survival of 1285 patients in Southeast Netherlands, 1984–1992. Eur J Cancer 2002; 38(3):409–413.
7. Altman E, Cadman E. An analysis of 1539 patients with cancer of unknown primary site. Cancer 1986; 57(1):120–124.
8. Abbruzzese JL, Abbruzzese MC, Hess KR, Raber MN, Lenzi R, Frost P. Unknown primary carcinoma: natural history and prognostic factors in 657 consecutive patients. J Clin Oncol 1994; 12(6):1272–1280.
9. Hess KR, Abbruzzese MC, Lenzi R, Raber MN, Abbruzzese JL. Classification and regression tree analysis of 1000 consecutive patients with unknown primary carcinoma. Clin Cancer Res 1999; 5(11):3403–3410.
10. Le Chevalier T, Cvitkovic E, Caille P, et al. Early metastatic cancer of unknown primary origin at presentation. A clinical study of 302 consecutive autopsied patients. Arch Intern Med 1988; 148(9):2035–2039.
11. Gamble AR, Bell JA, Ronan JE, Pearson D, Ellis IO. Use of tumor marker immunoreactivity to identify primary site of metastatic cancer [see comments]. Br Med J 1993; 306(6873):295–298.
12. DeYoung BR, Wick MR. Immunohistologic evaluation of metastatic carcinomas of unknown origin: an algorithmic approach. Semin Diagn Pathol 2000; 17(3):184–193.
13. Muir C. Cancer of unknown primary site. Cancer 1995; 75(suppl 1):353–356.
14. Blaszyk H, Hartmann A, Bjornsson J. Cancer of unknown primary: clinico-pathologic correlations. APMIS 2003; 111(12):1089–1094.
15. Levi F, Te VC, Erler G, Randimbison L, La Vecchia C. Epidemiology of unknown primary tumors. Eur J Cancer 2002; 38(13):1810–1812.
16. Krementz ET, Cerise EJ, Foster DS, Morgan LR, Jr. Metastases of undetermined source. Curr Probl Cancer 1979; 4(5):4–37.

17. Steckel RJ, Kagan AR. Metastatic tumors of unknown origin. Cancer 1991; 67(suppl 4):1242–1244.
18. European Network of Cancer Registries. Eurocim version 4.0. European Incidence Database V2.4. 730 Entity Dictionary (2003), Lyon 2001.
19. Daures JP, Tretarre B. Le cancer dans l'Herault 1999–2000. Mars 2003.
20. Parkin DM, Muir CS. Cancer incidence in five continents. Comparability and quality of data. IARC Sci Publ 1992; (120):45–173.
21. http://www.ikc.nl/vvik/kankerregistratie.
22. Leonard RJ, Nystrom JS. Diagnostic evaluation of patients with carcinoma of unknown primary tumor site. Semin Oncol 1993; 20(3):244–250.
23. Kirsten F, Chi CH, Leary JA, Ng AB, Hedley DW, Tattersall MH. Metastatic adeno or undifferentiated carcinoma from an unknown primary site—natural history and guidelines for identification of treatable subsets. Q J Med 1987; 62(238):143–161.
24. Didolkar MS, Fanous N, Elias EG, Moore RH. Metastatic carcinomas from occult primary tumors. A study of 254 patients. Ann Surg 1977; 186(5): 625–630.
25. Nystrom JS, Weiner JM, Heffelfinger-Juttner J, Irwin LE, Bateman JR, Wolf RM. Metastatic and histologic presentations in unknown primary cancer. Semin Oncol 1977; 4(1):53–58.
26. Hainsworth JD, Johnson DH, Greco FA. Poorly differentiated neuroendocrine carcinoma of unknown primary site. A newly recognized clinicopathologic entity. Ann Intern Med 1988; 109(5):364–371.
27. van de Wouw AJ, Jansen RL, Griffioen AW, Hillen HF. Clinical and immunohistochemical analysis of patients with unknown primary tumor. A search for prognostic factors in UPT. Anticancer Res 2004; 24(1):297–301.
28. Hamilton CS, Langlands AO. ACUPS (Adenocarcinoma of unknown primary site): a clinical and cost benefit analysis. Int J Radiat Oncol Biol Phys 1987; 13(10):1497–1503.
29. Stewart JF, Tattersall MH, Woods RL, Fox RM. Unknown primary adenocarcinoma: incidence of overinvestigation and natural history. Br Med J 1979; 1(6177):1530–1533.
30. Abbruzzese JL, Raber MN. Unknown primary. In: Abelhoff MD, Armitage JO, Lichter AS, Niederhuber JE, eds. Clinical Oncology. 1st ed. New York: Churchill Livingstone, 2001:1833–1845.
31. Culine S, Kramar A, Saghatchian M, et al. Development and validation of a prognostic model to predict the length of survival in patients with carcinomas of an unknown primary site. J Clin Oncol 2002; 20(24):4679–4683.
32. Gilbert HA, Kagan AR. Metastases: incidence, detection, and evaluation without histologic confirmation. In: Weiss L, ed. Fundamental Aspects of Metastasis. Amsterdam: North-Holland, 1976:385–405.
33. End Results Section, Biometry Branch National Cancer Institute. End results in cancer. Government Printing Office, 1972.
34. Abrams HL, Spiro R, Goldstein N. Metastases in carcinoma: analysis of 1000 autopsied cases. Cancer 1950; 3:74–85.
35. Mayordomo JI, Guerra JM, Guijarro C, et al. Neoplasms of unknown primary site: a clinicopathological study of autopsied patients. Tumori 1993; 79(5):321–324.

36. Fiore JJ, Kelsen DP, Gralla RJ, et al. Adenocarcinoma of unknown primary origin: treatment with vindesine and doxorubicin. Cancer Treat Rep 1985; 69(6):591–594.

37. Jordan WE III, Shildt RA. Adenocarcinoma of unknown primary site. The Brooke Army Medical Center Experience. Cancer 1985; 55(4):857–860.

38. Markman M. Metastatic adenocarcinoma of unknown primary site: analysis of 245 patients seen at the johns hopkins hospital from 1965–1979. Med Pediatr Oncol 1982; 10(6):569–574.

39. Hainsworth JD, Greco FA. Management of patients with cancer of unknown primary site. Oncology (Huntingt) 2000; 14(4):563–574.

40. Greco FA, Burris HA III, Litchy S, et al. Gemcitabine, carboplatin, and paclitaxel for patients with carcinoma of unknown primary site: a minnie pearl cancer Research Network Study. J Clin Oncol 2002; 20(6):1651–1656.

41. Greco FA, Erland JB, Morrissey LH, et al. Carcinoma of unknown primary site: phase II trials with docetaxel plus cisplatin or carboplatin. Ann Oncol 2000; 11(2):211–215.

42. Greco FA, Burris HA III, Erland JB, et al. Carcinoma of unknown primary site. Cancer 2000; 89(12):2655–2660.

43. Greco FA, Gray J, Burris HA III, Erland JB, Morrissey LH, Hainsworth JD. Taxane-based chemotherapy for patients with carcinoma of unknown primary site. Cancer J 2001; 7(3):203–212.

44. Hainsworth JD, Erland JB, Kalman LA, Schreeder MT, Greco FA. Carcinoma of unknown primary site: treatment with 1-hour paclitaxel, carboplatin, and extended-schedule etoposide. J Clin Oncol 1997; 15(6):2385–2393.

45. Lenzi R, Hess KR, Abbruzzese MC, Raber MN, Ordonez NG, Abbruzzese JL. Poorly differentiated carcinoma and poorly differentiated adenocarcinoma of unknown origin: favorable subsets of patients with unknown-primary carcinoma? J Clin Oncol 1997; 15(5):2056–2066.

46. Munoz A, Barcelo JR, Lopez-Vivanco G. Gemcitabine and docetaxel as front-line chemotherapy in patients with carcinoma of an unknown primary site. Cancer 2004; 101(3):653–654.

47. Pouessel D, Culine S, Becht C, et al. Gemcitabine and docetaxel as front-line chemotherapy in patients with carcinoma of an unknown primary site. Cancer 2004; 100(6):1257–1261.

48. Culine S, Lortholary A, Voigt JJ, et al. Cisplatin in combination with either gemcitabine or irinotecan in carcinomas of unknown primary site: results of a randomized phase II study-trial for the French Study Group on Carcinomas of Unknown Primary (GEFCAPI 01). J Clin Oncol 2003; 21(18):3479–3482.

49. Culine S, Fabbro M, Ychou M, Romieu G, Cupissol D, Pinguet F. Alternative bimonthly cycles of doxorubicin, cyclophosphamide, and etoposide, cisplatin with hematopoietic growth factor support in patients with carcinoma of unknown primary site. Cancer 2002; 94(3):840–846.

50. van der Gaast A, Verweij J, Planting AS, Hop WC, Stoter G. Simple prognostic model to predict survival in patients with undifferentiated carcinoma of unknown primary site. J Clin Oncol 1995; 13(7):1720–1725.

DIAGNOSTIC EVALUATION IN CARCINOMAS OF UNKNOWN
PRIMARY SITE: WHAT SHALL WE DO AND WHEN SHALL
WE STOP SEEKING THE PRIMARY SITE?

—————————————— **2** ——————————————

Radiographic Studies, Endoscopy, and Serum Tumor Markers in the Diagnostic Evaluation of Carcinomas of Unknown Primary Site

Gauri R. Varadhachary and Renato Lenzi

*Department of Gastrointestinal Medical Oncology, The University of Texas
M.D. Anderson Cancer Center, Houston, Texas, U.S.A.*

INTRODUCTION

The identification of a primary site of origin is the initial step in the formulation of the plan of treatment and in the determination of prognosis for oncology patients. When metastatic disease is documented in the absence of a clear primary site, a careful selection of the diagnostic tests to be performed is of paramount importance to maximize the chances of identifying the primary tumor and to minimize treatment delay, patient risk, inconvenience, and costs associated with a lengthy and redundant work-up.

For some of the patients presenting with metastatic disease in the absence of a clear primary site (occult primary), re-evaluation of material obtained at biopsy may reveal a specific histology and thus provide the diagnosis; in the majority of patients, however, the identification of the primary tumor requires a combination of pathology review, laboratory studies, and imaging and/or endoscopic studies (1). When pathology evaluation alone is not sufficient to determine the primary, identification of the site of origin using available diagnostic modalities is arduous, and in fact it is impossible in the majority of these patients.

The underlying causes of this difficulty are not well defined, but certain biological aspects of carcinomas of unknown primary may offer clues to possible contributing factors (2). Observations of the patterns of metastatic disease in patients presenting with occult primary tumors that were eventually discovered at autopsy suggest that epidemiology, sites of metastatic spread, and histologic characteristics may be unusual in these patients. Thus, Nystrom et al. (3) described a higher than expected incidence of lung cancer in female patients, accompanied by a lower than expected (4%) incidence of bone metastasis; patients with colon and pancreas cancer had an unusually high (30%) incidence of bone metastasis and patients with prostate cancer had an unusually high incidence of lung and liver metastases (75% and 50%).

It has been hypothesized that tumors presenting with metastatic disease in the absence of a clearly identifiable primary may have a distinct malignant phenotype with early metastatic potential that does not conform to a pattern of sustained local growth and spread by regional and distant metastases (4). As a result of biological characteristics such as angiogenic incompetency, the primary tumor may never reach a size detectable by the commonly used diagnostic imaging modalities [chest X ray, computed axial tomography (CT), or endoscopy] or disappear after seeding metastasis that may eventually acquire an angiogenic phenotype (5) and grow to reach the threshold of clinical detection. Hillen et al. (6) tested the hypothesis that increased microvessel density (MVD) in carcinomas of unknown primary (CUP) metastasis might differentiate them from those of known primaries and result in early and widespread metastasis. Their comparitive study of metastatic liver lesions from CUP with metastatic liver lesions from colon and breast cancer, however, showed a similar MVD. Observations in human cancer cell lines (7) and in human subjects (8) support the notion that the ability to metastasize can be acquired early during the process of tumorigenesis; in breast cancer, molecular profiles predicting development of metastatic disease and poor survival have been identified early in the disease (9), and it is conceivable that for some patients this may result in the development nearly synchronous metastatic and primary lesions obfuscating the expected pattern of a larger primary and smaller metastatic lesions. These scenarios have been invoked in an attempt to explain why, despite the technical advances in laboratory and imaging techniques, the diagnostic evaluation of patients presenting with an occult primary remains challenging, with an overall rate of identification of the primary remaining between 20% and 30% (1,10).

Factors potentially affecting the results of studies of diagnostic strategies for the evaluation of patients presenting with an occult primary include regional differences in the prevalence of certain types of cancer, diagnostic modalities available at the time the patients were evaluated, referral patterns, the extent of evaluation prior to study entry, and the definition of the criteria to be met in order to classify a primary as diagnosed. Earlier studies conducted before the widespread use of CT scanning, a diagnostic instrument with high relative yield in this patient population, are also those with the majority of available data derived from postmortem evaluation, while more recent studies on patients populations extensively investigated by CT reflect the sharp decrease in the number of postmortem evaluations performed in more recent years, complicating to some extent comparisons of data obtained at different time periods. Most of the available studies have been retrospective, and many of the parameters used for patient selection have varied among different groups of investigators. It is, however, apparent from the literature that the majority of the patients presenting with an occult primary remain undiagnosed regardless of the exhaustiveness of the work-up, and that a focused approach aimed at detecting those primary cancers for which effective treatment is available is generally preferred.

In this chapter we review the diagnostic yield and the indications of chest X ray, CT, and endoscopic studies in the evaluation of patients with occult primary cancer, focusing on those not belonging in defined "favorable" clinicopathological subgroups (11). Because of the frequent inclusion of the determination of tumor markers levels in the initial work-up of patients with an occult primary and of the not infrequent triggering of additional diagnostic tests based on those results, we also briefly review the role of certain common tumor markers in the diagnostic evaluation.

CHEST X RAY

Chest X ray has historically been part of the routine evaluation of patients with an occult primary, reflecting the frequent involvement of the lungs in metastatic disease and the fact that lung cancer is among the most commonly detected primary cancers (1). If malignant lesions are visible on chest X ray, this is a simple follow-up test to evaluate the status of the disease. Given its limited resolution, many patients are also routinely studied with a CT scan of the chest (12).

Nystrom et al. described in detail some of the challenges in the correct classification of malignant lung lesions as primary or metastatic based on their appearance on chest X ray. In their series of 266 occult primary patients, the majority were evaluated with history and physical examination, chemistry profile, urinalysis, proctosigmoidodscopy, upper gastrointestinal (GI) tract contrast radiographic study, single-contrast barium enema, bone survey, liver scan, chest X ray, intravenous pyelogram, and mammogram (in women). The diagnostic yield of this evaluation was of 22 primary cancers detected in 136 patients who did not have an autopsy. Of the 130 patients who had an autopsy, a primary cancer was eventually detected in 107 patients. Review of the chest roentgenograms of 64 patients with verified primary (27) or metastatic (37) lung lesions identified five patterns: single lung mass, malignant pleural effusions, multiple nodules, nodal disease, and infiltrative lesions (13). Of these, the presence of a single lung mass, pleural effusion, or regional nodal disease were not helpful in distinguishing primary lung cancer from metastatic disease, while the presence of multiple nodules and infiltrative lesions was more frequently associated with a diagnosis of metastatic disease of the lungs than with primary lung cancer (13). Le Chevalier et al. (14) studied 302 consecutive autopsied patients who presented with an occult primary and the primary site identified antemortem in 27% of the patients and postmortem in 57% of the patients. In 16% of the cases , the site remained unidentified. The most frequent sites were pancreas (26.5%), lung (17.2%), kidney (4.6%), and colorectum (3.6%). The chest X ray was abnormal in 184 cases, and of those 96 cases were deemed to have primary lung cancer. However, a diagnosis of primary lung cancer was confirmed at autopsy in only 36 cases.

In a retrospective study of 32 patients with an occult primary presenting with brain metastasis (15) and who had both chest X ray and chest CT, both tests were negative in one patient (who was eventually diagnosed with breast cancer). All other patients were diagnosed with primary lung cancer. Of those, 19 patients had positive chest X rays and chest CTs, and 12 had a positive CT chest with a negative or indeterminate chest X ray. The mean size of the primary tumor was significantly larger in the patients with a positive chest X ray (4.2 vs. 2.5 cm, $P < 0.1$).

COMPUTED AXIAL TOMOGRAPHY

Karsell et al. (16) evaluated the diagnostic yield of CT while evaluating patients referred for scanning with a diagnosis of metastatic cancer of unknown primary source. Of 98 study patients, 85 had an abdominal CT, 9 had a chest CT only, and 4 had both tests. A primary cancer was identified and confirmed histologically in 30 patients. In one patient the vascular pattern at angiography was deemed to confirm the CT diagnosis of primary hepatoma. In three cases, the CT findings were subsequently proved not to represent a malignancy and were considered false positives. In addition, in 23 patients the CT scan demonstrated metastatic lesions, which were undetected before the test in 9 patients. In those patients, 19 primaries were never detected and 4 were located in areas not included in the CT field. In 41 patients, the CT scan did not reveal either primary or metastatic disease. Of these cases, 12 were confirmed as negative (in 10 the primary was diagnosed at a site not included in the CT field and in 2 patients only benign disease was detected). In 16 patients a primary tumor was never identified. There were 13 false negative results (a primary tumor was later detected within the imaged field). Of these, in one case a primary carcinoid tumor was missed because only the upper portion of the abdomen was included in the CT. In six patients, in retrospect the primary and/or strong clues to its present clues were imaged on CT but were not recognized as such (retroperitoneal mass of embryonal cell carcinoma, pancreatic primary in a background of postsurgical changes from pseudocystojejunostomy, two ovarian cancers on a background of large volume ascites, gallbladder dilatation secondary to primary carcinoma of the gallbladder, and small soft tissue mass corresponding to an annular colon carcinoma causing distal filling defect). Other primary tumors that went undiagnosed by CT (three prostatic, one ileal, and two pancreatic primaries) were of a size below the resolution of the technique. In 23 patients, the CT scan demonstrated metastatic lesions only; in nine of those patients, those lesions had escaped detection by other diagnostic means. Based on these results, the authors advocated the use of CT scan for the evaluation of patients presenting with an occult primary tumor, based on symptoms, the results of physical exam, pathology review, and sites of metastases.

McMillan et al. (17) studied a population of 75 patients with occult primary cancer referred for CT evaluation. Patients with a history of a prior known malignancy, squamous carcinoma in cervical lymph nodes, repeat histological evaluation revealing lymphoma or multiple myeloma, isolated lung lesions on chest X ray subsequently determined to represent primary lung cancer, and two patients with obvious primary tumors that were over-looked in the initial evaluation were excluded. The remaining 46 patients all had histologically proved metastatic adenocarcinomas or poorly differen-tiated carcinomas. Chest radiography and abdominal CT were performed in all patients. Pelvic CT or ultrasound were performed in 40 patients. Thirty-three patients had an upper GI series, and thirty-four had a barium enema. Eleven patients had an exploratory laparotomy, nine had a broncho-scopy, three a gastroscopy, and one a colonoscopy. Autopsies were per-formed in five. Thirteen of forty-six abdominal CT scans, two of thirteen pelvic CT scans, and one of seven chest CT scans performed were diagnostic of the primary. Thus, CT scanning was diagnostic in 34.8% of patients. Abdominal CT scan failed to detect primary colon cancer in one patient. CT scans were negative in 25 patients who remained undiagnosed. Four patients were diagnosed with primaries at sites not studied by CT. In 30 patients (65%), CT imaging showed metastasis, which was not detected previously. CT proved superior to sonography and contrast studies of the urinary and GI tracts. The authors recommended the inclusion of CT of the abdomen and CT of the pelvis/ultrasound as part of the routine evalua-tion of patients with occult primary carcinoma, based on the potential of these tests to increase the rate of detection of the primary, and to provide information on the extent of the disease. Chest CT in this study was not considered to provide sufficient additional diagnostic information to recom-mend its routine use as a baseline diagnostic test.

Abbruzzese et al. (1) studied 879 patients referred with a diagnosis of metastatic cancer of unknown primary, and evaluated the use of a limited initial diagnostic approach that included review of biopsy material, history and phy-sical exam, CBC, chemistry survey, chest X ray, and CT of abdomen and pelvis. Women were additionally evaluated with a mammogram; prostate specific antigen, beta human chorionic gonadotropin, and α-fetoprotein (AFP) levels were obtained in men. Additional studies were done only if indicated by abnormal findings detected during the above evaluation. Patients with a referral diagnosis of carcinoma, who upon review were determined to have a different type of cancer of noncarcinoma histology (such as lymphoma, leukemia, melanoma, sarcoma), were considered to have their primary detected upon recognition of the specific histology and additional imaging studies were not required for the purpose of categorizing the primary as diagnosed. Of these cases 180 primary tumors were identified (one patient had two primaries), and in 58 of these the diagnosis was made on the basis of specific histologic features alone. The remainder of the malignancies were of common epithelial histology (carcinomas devoid of characteristic identifying features) and required additional testing to determine the diagnosis. For patients with carcinomas, the three most common diagnoses were lung (27), pancreas (21), and colorectal (11), followed by kidney (9), breast (8), stomach (8), ovary (6), liver (6), esophagus (5), mesothelioma (4), prostate (4), and "other" (32). CT of the abdomen was diagnostic in 86% of the pancreatic cancers cases and in 36% of the colorectal patients. CT of the chest and bronchoscopy identified 74% and 26% of the lung cancers detected, respectively. Overall, CT scan was the diagnostic modality in 55% of the primary tumors detected.

CONTRAST STUDIES OF THE GI TRACT AND ENDOSCOPIC PROCEDURES

Earlier studies of patients presenting with an occult primary relied heavily on contrast roentgenographic studies of the GI tract and on endoscopic procedures. Data reported in some of those studies have included the results of postmortem evaluations, and provide a useful perspective on the distribution of primary type in those patients. In the series reported by Nystrom et al. of 218 patients who underwent contrast radiographic studies of the upper GI tract, eight were correctly diagnosed with a primary (gastric cancer), and six had false positive diagnoses of gastric cancer that were disproven at autopsy. Of 198 patients who underwent barium enema, 17 were initially diagnosed with colorectal cancer; eight of those diagnoses were determined to be false positives at autopsy. The rate of false negative results could not be established in this study because 99 study patients whose primary was not detected after clinical evaluation did not undergo autopsy. Given the low diagnostic yield and the high percentage of false positives, the authors concluded that the use of these tests should be limited to patients with specific indications such as hemoccult positive stool.

In 150 of the patients studied by LeChevalier et al. (14), a contrast study of the upper GI tract was obtained. In 28 of those patients the test was deemed to show cancer; in 6 the primary site (gastric, 5; esophageal, 1) was confirmed at autopsy. In the same study, 105 patients had barium enemas, and 8 were interpreted as showing cancerous involvement. One false positive and two false-negative (sigmoid cancer) results were observed. The true positive diagnoses were three cecal, two rectal cancers, and two instances of local involvement by pancreas cancer.

Esophageal and gastric endoscopy was performed in 35 patients, with abnormal findings in 12 (gastric primary, 3; gastric metastasis from pancreas primary, 1; esophageal metastasis from pancreatic cancer, 2; esophageal metastasis from prostatic cancer, 1; esophageal direct involvement from lung cancer, 2; extrinsic compression, 3). There were three false negative results. Proctoscopy was done in 28 patients, with abnormal findings in 3 (rectal carcinoma, 2; ureteral carcinoma metastasis, 1). Bronchoscopy was done in 105 patients and was prompted by imaging or pathology findings. While results were "abnormal" for malignancy in 73, only 19 patients were confirmed to have primary lung cancer at autopsy.

In the series reported by McMillan et al., contrast studies of the upper GI tract were performed in 33 patients, and were interpreted as normal; one of those patients was subsequently diagnosed with gastric cancer. Barium enema was performed in 34 patients. Of those, one was diagnosed with sigmoid carcinoma, which was confirmed at surgery. Gastroscopy was performed on three patients, colonoscopy on one patient, and bronchoscopy on nine patients. No primary was diagnosed by endoscopy; one false negative result was determined in these studies (bronchogenic carcinoma).

Patients with Metastatic Liver Involvement

Given the propensity of GI primary tumors to metastasize to the liver, it would be expected that a higher percentage of those primaries would be diagnosed in patients with metastatic liver involvement.

A study by Ayob et al. focused on patients referred for evaluation of an occult primary, who had metastatic liver lesions. Of 1522 consecutive patients, 500 had liver metastasis. In 27% of those, a primary site was identified using a limited diagnostic evaluation (10). The most common primary (25 patients) was lung, followed by colorectal (23 patients), pancreas (22 patients), liver (13 patients), melanoma (9 patients), breast (8 patients), gastric (7 patients), and other primary sites with five patients or less each. The diagnostic study with the highest yield was CT of the abdomen/pelvis (40 patients diagnosed), followed by pathology evaluation (37), chest X ray (17), esophago-gastro-duodenoscopy (6), colonoscopy (5), barium enema (8), and CT chest (4). Upper GI and bronchoscopy were diagnostic in three and two patients, respectively, and other modalities were diagnostic in two or less each (two patients were diagnosed at autopsy). The conclusion that can be drawn from these studies is that in the general population of patients with an occult primary carcinoma, GI contrast studies and endoscopy should be limited to patients with specific symptoms or abnormalities detected in the initial work-up (1). In patients presenting with liver metastasis, however, the prevalence of colorectal primaries appears to be higher than in the overall population of patients with occult primaries. As the prognosis of patients with colorectal cancer in the metastatic stage has improved with the recent introduction of more effective chemotherapy regimens (18), it is important to diagnose this condition, and colonoscopy should be considered even in the absence of specific symptoms, particularly if the evaluation of biopsy material is suggestive of a colorectal primary (e.g., adenocarcinoma histology with cytokeratin 7 negative and cytokeratin 20 positive by immunohistochemistry) (19).

SERUM TUMOR MARKERS

In our practice we frequently encounter patients who prior to their referral for evaluation of an occult primary have undergone specific diagnostic tests that were requested solely because of the elevation of certain tumor markers [such as colonoscopy performed on the basis of an elevated carcinoembryonic antigen (CEA)]. The available evidence, however, does not support a practical diagnostic value for the elevation of clinically available serum tumor markers.

In a study by Koch and McPherson (20), 34 patients presenting with an occult primary were studied and compared with 542 patients with known primaries and at least one site of metastatic disease. All patients had CEA levels measured. The primary of origin was eventually detected in all occult primary patients at autopsy (30 patients), at surgery (3 patients), or became apparent after prolonged follow-up (1 patient). Six patients with noncarcinomatous histology were included; none of those had a CEA level of >10 ng/mL. In the remaining patients, levels of CEA ≤10 ng/mL were not correlated with any specific primary tumor of origin and were not deemed to be clinically useful. On the basis of the observations in patients presenting with a known primary, levels >10 ng/mL were hypothesized to favor a primary of GI, respiratory tract, breast, or ovarian (mucinous) origin. For the 10 patients with CEA levels >10 ng/mL, the corresponding diagnoses were lung (five patients), pancreas (two patients), bile duct (one patient), and ovary (two patients). The range of diagnostic possibilities associated to the level of CEA elevation remained, however, large and of limited relevance to diagnosis or treatment.

In a study by Le Chevalier et al. (14), tumor marker studies of CEA, β-human chorionic gonadotropin (β-HCG), and AFP were done in 15 patients each and were deemed of no diagnostic significance. The prostatic fraction of acid phosphatase was also studied in 45 patients and was elevated in three; none of the patients was diagnosed with prostate cancer at autopsy, and of the six patients diagnosed with prostate cancer at autopsy none had elevated levels of acid phosphatase levels.

In a study of 147 consecutive occult primary patients studied at M.D. Anderson Cancer Center, 41 had a CEA level higher than 10 ng/mL; this information did not contribute to the diagnosis of a primary site (21).

Pavlidis et al. evaluated CEA, CA 19-9, CA 15-3, CA 125, β-HCG, and AFP in 85 patients with CUP. Tumor histology was undifferentiated carcinoma in 65% of the patients and adenocarcinoma in 35%. Metastatic sites were one in 32%, two in 35%, and three or more in 33% of the patients. Sex distribution was 29 males and 56 females. CEA levels were elevated in 52%, CA 19-9 in 63%, CA 15-3 in 60%, CA 125 in 69%, β-HCG in 44%, and AFP in 17%. Mean values of CA 19-9 and CA-125 levels were significantly different in patients with two compared with one metastatic site. CEA and CA 19-9 were significantly higher in patients with liver metastasis compared with patients with lymph node metastasis. None of the markers were predictors of response to chemotherapy and there was no significant correlation for any of the markers with survival. The study results did not support any utility of the tumor markers studied in the diagnosis or estimate of prognosis in CUP patients (20).

As part of a study of the clinical outcomes of CUP patients with poorly differentiated carcinoma histology, the correlation of elevated β-HCG, AFP, and survival were studied by Lenzi et al. (22) to obtain some insight into the possibility that elevation of these tumor markers in patients with poorly differentiated carcinoma histology might identify patients with better overall treatment response and prognosis. In 74 and 54, respectively, of 337 patients with poorly differentiated histology, β-HCG and AFP levels were measured; in 51 patients both measurements were available. There was no correlation between the levels of the two markers. When survival of the patients with measured levels of β-HCG and AFP was studied, 21 patients with AFP levels < 2.8 ng/mL and β-HCG levels < 3.4 mIU/mL had a median survival of 17 months, the 13 patients with AFP levels >2.8 ng/ mL and HCG < 3.4 mIU/mL had a median survival of six months, and 17 patients with β-HCG levels >3.4 mIU/mL had a median survival of five months.

The levels of these markers in the general population of occult primary patients with poorly differentiated carcinomas therefore did not appear to have prognostic value, although they may be useful in patients with other clinical characteristics of the extragonadal germ cell syndrome (23).

SURVIVAL PATTERNS AND THEIR EFFECT ON DIAGNOSTIC STRATEGIES IN PATIENTS PRESENTING WITH OCCULT PRIMARY CANCER

The diagnostic evaluation of patients presenting with an occult primary is complex, time-consuming, expensive, and some of the diagnostic procedures involved carry a significant risk for the patient.

A potential advantage might exist from identifying a primary that could be amenable to local treatment, avoiding potentially serious local complications (e.g., bowel obstruction or bleeding from a GI primary). For some patients there may be a psychological benefit in removing the uncertainty regarding the diagnosis. However, an extensive work-up would be difficult to justify without evidence that detecting the primary may allow for effective interventions on the overall disease process resulting in a more favorable outcome (24). In an asymptomatic patient with metastatic disease, the detection of a small primary tumor is generally unlikely to affect the clinical course unless effective treatment is available for that particular diagnosis that would not have been used, had the nature of the primary remained unknown. The potential impact of different diagnostic outcomes on choice of treatment and survival therefore needs to be considered in the planning of a diagnostic strategy and improvements in the efficacy of available treatment for certain primary tumors resulting in more favorable outcomes need to be considered in the formulation of diagnostic strategies for occult primary tumors.

In a study by Abbruzzese et al. (11), survival of 179 patients who after evaluation were diagnosed with a specific primary site was statistically significantly longer than that of the 657 patients who remained undiagnosed (15 months; CI, 11–20 months and 11 months; CI 10–12 months). Further analysis of survival duration by primary site provided information regarding the contribution of different subsets of patients to the overall outcome of the group. The 39 patients who were diagnosed with lymphoma, melanoma, or sarcoma had significantly longer median survival (20 months; 95% CI, 13–31 months, $P = 0.0010$) compared with the patients with CUP (13 months; 95% CI, 8–17 months). Lymphoma patients had the longest survival in that group and accounted for most of the longer survival duration. For these patients histological evaluation of biopsy material was the diagnostic modality, and CT and other imaging studies had a secondary role. Of the patients diagnosed with primaries of common epithelial histology, who were mostly diagnosed by a combination of pathology evaluation and imaging studies, the survival of patients with primary lung cancer, pancreatic cancer, and colon cancer did not differ from that of CUP patients, probably reflecting the limited efficacy of available treatment for those primary cancers in the metastatic stage at the time of the study.

The largest contribution to the longer overall survival of patients with diagnosed primary tumors of common epithelial histology was from patients with primary ovarian and breast cancers (6 and 8, respectively). In this study, CT scan was the diagnostic modality in 55 of 122 patients with common epithelial histology, but only five of the patients diagnosed by CT (four with ovarian and one with head and neck cancer) had cancers that were considered to be highly treatable at the time.

Primary cancers diagnosed by endoscopy were not associated with longer survival. Therefore, endoscopic evaluation was recommended only to investigate abnormalities detected during routine work-up. The availability of more sensitive and specific immunohistochemical reagents may provide additional guidance in the selection of patients for endoscopic procedures that have a relatively low yield when performed based solely on clinical and radiographic criteria (25); thus bronchoscopy could be considered based on morphology and immunohistochemistry, consistent with a lung primary (26).

Improvement in the survival of patients with common epithelial cancers in the metastatic stage (such as the recent improvement of survival duration achieved in patients with advanced colorectal cancer) (27) have changed the expected outcome of therapy targeted to certain common epithelial cancers, and it seems prudent to adjust the diagnostic strategy to more aggressively pursue those diagnoses, as more primary types in the metastatic stage are added to the list of potentially highly treatable cancers. Whether the improved outcomes of patients presenting with an obvious primary in an advanced stage (e.g., colorectal) do indeed also apply to patients with the same condition presenting as an occult primary seems reasonable to expect based on current experience with ovarian (28), breast (29), and head and neck cancers (30), but will need to be investigated in future studies.

CONCLUSION AND FUTURE DIRECTIONS

In early studies of patients presenting with CUP, overall survival durations as short as five months were not uncommon, regardless of whether a primary was detected or not (14); in more recent series, median survival has approximately doubled for the overall population of CUP patients (31), and even longer survival durations have been reported for patients eventually diagnosed with certain types of primary tumors (1). The strategy for the diagnostic evaluation of patients presenting with an occult primary has continued to evolve under the pressure of strong determinants of change such as the availability of more sophisticated diagnostic techniques and therapeutic advances in the treatment of certain primary tumors that make their identification relevant to the goal of achieving better treatment outcomes (such as higher rates of response and longer survival duration).

Abdominal/chest CT scanning remains a mainstay of the diagnostic evaluation of patients with occult primary, because of the relatively high rate of detection of the primary of origin and of the information provided on the location and extent of metastatic disease that are of independent predictor of prognosis (32). The role of endoscopy, established in the evaluation of patients with squamous cell carcinoma of high and/or mid-neck nodal metastsis (33), remains incompletely defined in patients not belonging in this "favorable" clinicopathological subgroup, but a more frequent use of this diagnostic modality appears justified in patients with clinicopathological characteristics suggesting a possible colorectal primary, given the advances in the treatment of this condition.

As outcomes continue to improve for patients with common epithelial cancers in the metastatic stage, the list of primary diagnosis that is important to determine when evaluating patients with an occult primary can be expected to expand even further, making the development of more effective diagnostic strategies necessary. Advances can therefore be expected from the rational integration of additional imaging techniques such as magnetic resonance imaging and positron emission tomography/CT scanning into the evaluation of occult primary patients, and by the definition of new criteria for the appropriate use of diagnostic procedures such as endoscopy of the GI and respiratory tracts. Advances in the laboratory diagnosis such as the availability of more reliable immunohistochemistry reagent and in the near future of gene profiling will also require a periodical re-evaluation of the indications for imaging and endoscopic procedures in the diagnosis of these patients.

REFERENCES

1. Abbruzzese JL, Abbruzzese MC, Lenzi R, Hess KR, Raber MN. Analysis of a diagnostic strategy for patients with suspected tumors of unknown origin. J Clin Oncol 1995; 13(8):2094–2103.
2. Hillen HF. Unknown primary tumours. Postgrad Med J 2000; 76(901):690–693.
3. Nystrom JS, Weiner JM, Heffelfinger-Juttner J, Irwin LE, Bateman JR, Wolf RM. Metastatic and histologic presentations in unknown primary cancer. Semin Oncol 1977; 4(1):53–58.
4. Abbruzzese JL, Lenzi R, Raber MN, Pathak S, Frost P. The biology of unknown primary tumors. Semin Oncol 1993; 20(3):238–243.
5. Naresh KN. Do metastatic tumours from an unknown primary reflect angiogenic incompetence of the tumour at the primary site?—a hypothesis. Med Hypotheses 2002; 59(3):357–360.
6. Hillen HF, Hak LE, Joosten-Achjanie SR, Arends JW. Microvessel density in unknown primary tumors. Int J Cancer 1997; 74(1):81–85.
7. Kang Y, Siegel PM, Shu W, et al. A multigenic program mediating breast cancer metastasis to bone. Cancer Cell 2003; 3(6):537–549.
8. Van't Veer LJ, Weigelt B. Road map to metastasis. Nat Med 2003; 9(8):999–1000.
9. van de Vijver MJ, He YD, van't Veer LJ, et al. A gene-expression signature as a predictor of survival in breast cancer. N Engl J Med 2002; 347(25):1999–2009.
10. Ayoub JP, Hess KR, Abbruzzese MC, Lenzi R, Raber MN, Abbruzzese JL. Unknown primary tumors metastatic to liver. J Clin Oncol 1998; 16(6):2105–2112.
11. Abbruzzese JL, Abbruzzese MC, Hess KR, Raber MN, Lenzi R, Frost P. Unknown primary carcinoma: natural history and prognostic factors in 657 consecutive patients. J Clin Oncol 1994; 12(6):1272–1280.
12. Culine S, Fabbro M, Ychou M, Romieu G, Cupissol D, Pinguet F. Alternative bimonthly cycles of doxorubicin, cyclophosphamide, and etoposide, cisplatin with hematopoietic growth factor support in patients with carcinoma of unknown primary site. Cancer 2002; 94(3):840–846.

13. Nystrom JS, Weiner JM, Wolf RM, Bateman JR, Viola MV. Identifying the primary site in metastatic cancer of unknown origin. Inadequacy of roentgenographic procedures. JAMA 1979; 241(4):381–383.
14. Le Chevalier T, Cvitkovic E, Caille P, et al. Early metastatic cancer of unknown primary origin at presentation. A clinical study of 302 consecutive autopsied patients. Arch Intern Med 1988; 148(9):2035–2039.
15. Latief KH, White CS, Protopapas Z, Attar S, Krasna MJ. Search for a primary lung neoplasm in patients with brain metastasis: is the chest radiograph sufficient? Am J Roentgenol 1997; 168(5):1339–1344.
16. Karsell PR, Sheedy PF II, O'Connell MJ. Computed tomography in search of cancer of unknown origin. JAMA 1982; 248(3):340–343.
17. McMillan JH, Levine E, Stephens RH. Computed tomography in the evaluation of metastatic adenocarcinoma from an unknown primary site. A retrospective study. Radiology 1982; 143(1):143–146.
18. Grothey A, Sargent D, Goldberg RM, Schmoll HJ. Survival of patients with advanced colorectal cancer improves with the availability of fluorouracil-leucovorin, irinotecan, and oxaliplatin in the course of treatment. J Clin Oncol 2004; 22(7):1209–1214.
19. Tot T. Adenocarcinomas metastatic to the liver: the value of cytokeratins 20 and 7 in the search for unknown primary tumors. Cancer 1999; 85(1):171–177.
20. Koch M, McPherson TA. Carcinoembryonic antigen levels as an indicator of the primary site in metastatic disease of unknown origin. Cancer 1981; 48(5):1242–1244.
21. Varadhachary GR, Abbruzzese JL, Lenzi R. Diagnostic strategies for unknown primary cancer. Cancer 2004; 100(9):1776–1785.
22. Lenzi R, Hess KR, Abbruzzese MC, Raber MN, Ordonez NG, Abbruzzese JL. Poorly differentiated carcinoma and poorly differentiated adenocarcinoma of unknown origin: favorable subsets of patients with unknown-primary carcinoma? J Clin Oncol 1997; 15(5):2056–2066.
23. Richardson RL, Schoumacher RA, Fer MF, et al. The unrecognized extragonadal germ cell cancer syndrome. Ann Intern Med 1981; 94(2):181–186.
24. Fizazi K, Culine S. Metastatic carcinoma of unknown origin. Bull Cancer 1998; 85(7):609–617.
25. Edwards FH, Schaefer PS, Callahan S, Graeber GM, Albus RA. Bayesian statistical theory in the preoperative diagnosis of pulmonary lesions. Chest 1987; 92(5):888–891.
26. Jerome Marson V, Mazieres J, Groussard O, et al. Expression of TTF-1 and cytokeratins in primary and secondary epithelial lung tumours: correlation with histological type and grade. Histopathology 2004; 45(2):125–134.
27. Meyerhardt JA, Mayer RJ. Systemic therapy for colorectal cancer. N Engl J Med 2005; 352(5):476–487.
28. Strnad CM, Grosh WW, Baxter J, et al. Peritoneal carcinomatosis of unknown primary site in women. A distinctive subset of adenocarcinoma. Ann Intern Med 1989; 111(3):213–217.
29. Vlastos G, Jean ME, Mirza AN, et al. Feasibility of breast preservation in the treatment of occult primary carcinoma presenting with axillary metastases. Ann Surg Oncol 2001; 8(5):425–431.

30. Mendenhall WM, Mancuso AA, Amdur RJ, Stringer SP, Villaret DB, Cassisi NJ. Squamous cell carcinoma metastatic to the neck from an unknown head and neck primary site. Am J Otolaryngol 2001; 22(4):261–267.
31. Hainsworth JD, Erland JB, Kalman LA, Schreeder MT, Greco FA. Carcinoma of unknown primary site: treatment with 1-hour paclitaxel, carboplatin, and extended-schedule etoposide. J Clin Oncol 1997; 15(6):2385–2393.
32. Hess KR, Abbruzzese MC, Lenzi R, Raber MN, Abbruzzese JL. Classification and regression tree analysis of 1000 consecutive patients with unknown primary carcinoma. Clin Cancer Res 1999; 5(11):3403–3410.
33. Bugat R, Bataillard A, Lesimple T, et al. Summary of the standards, options and recommendations for the management of patients with carcinoma of unknown primary site (2002). Br J Cancer 2003; 89(suppl 1):S59–S66.

3

The Advent of Immunohistochemistry in Carcinoma of Unknown Primary Site: A Major Progress

Jean-Jacques Voigt

Department of Pathology, Institut Claudius Regaud, Toulouse, France

Marie-Christine Mathieu

Department of Pathology, Institut Gustave Roussy, Villejuif, France

Frédéric Bibeau

Department of Pathology, Centre Val d'Aurelle, Montpellier, France

INTRODUCTION

Carcinoma of unknown primary (CUP) is a metastatic malignant epithelial tumor (1). Lymph nodes are the most frequent sites (about one-third of the cases) with the anatomical site being, in order of frequency, cervical, mediastinal, retroperitoneal, and inguinal. Other major sites of CUPs include the liver, the bones, the lungs, and the brain. CUP belongs to a heterogeneous entity owing to the variety of histopathological types and sites of metastases. The primary site remains unknown in more than 25% of patients. Prognosis is usually poor with a median survival time of only few months (2–4).

However, because therapy is a challenge in CUP and because subsets with favorable prognosis and/or a specific treatment have been identified (see Chapter 7), diagnostic accuracy is of paramount importance. Thus, differential diagnosis with primary carcinomas and other types of tumors (lymphoma, germ cell tumor, melanoma, sarcoma, etc.) is of major importance.

Immunohistochemistry is therefore an indispensable tool (5–7). Currently, the role of the pathologist is to determine the histopathological type rather than the origin of the primary tumor in view of a suitable therapy based on clinical, morphological, and phenotypic data. Strategies for this practical approach are proposed in two algorithms (Figs. 1 and 2). Abbreviations and their meanings are listed in Table 1 (8–10).

METHODS

Clinical Data

Clinical, radiological, and biological data are very important references for the pathological management of the tumor. Therefore, it is recommended that a summary of the clinical case is provided to the pathologist, and/or that the treating physician and the pathologist discuss the case together.

Management of Samples

In general, the small size of the samples obtained by core tissue biopsy justify careful management of the tumoral tissue. Necrosis, artefact of fixation, and crush can reduce the volume of interpretable tissue. When available, fresh tissue should be stored for cryopreservation, in view of molecular biology. Some special stainings can be useful to reveal mucus, bile, or melanin. Samples should be adequately fixed in formalin or AFA (acetic acid, formaldehyde, alcohol). The standard staining that allows microscopic examination is hematoxylin and eosin.

Indeed, morphology constitutes the basis for diagnosis, but it may be usefully supplemented by immunohistochemistry. This investigation is a powerful technique to obtain additional diagnostic information. However, one should keep in mind that a valid sample and a relevant panel of antibodies are needed for specificity and sensitivity. Even the most specific antibodies (as PSA) are not entirely site-specific. For more detailed information on immunohistochemistry, standard textbooks are available (7). Moreover, strict quality assurance procedures have been developed.

It is of great interest to bear in mind Gown's laws of immunohistochemistry (11):

1. There is no perfect marker for anything.
2. There is no perfect fixative for everything.
3. If everything is positive, nothing is positive.
4. All that turns brown (black, red, etc.) is not positive.
5. Tissue will fall off the slide corresponding to the most critical antibody in any given immunohistochemical run.
6. The diagnostic power of any immunohistochemical preparation is no greater than the wisdom of the pathologist interpreting it.

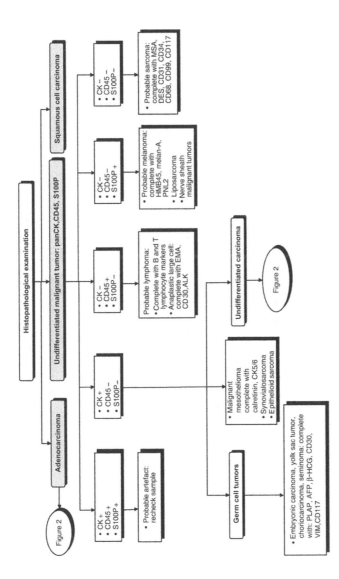

Figure 1   Algorithm for histopathological diagnosis of carcinoma of unknown primary site. *Source*: From Ref. 8.

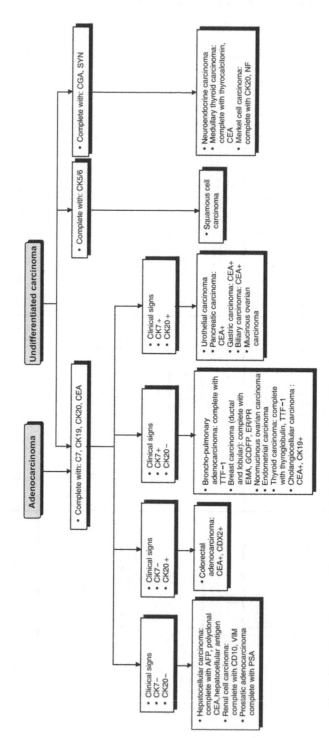

Figure 2 Algorithm for histopathological diagnosis of undifferentiated carcinoma or adenocarcinoma. *Source:* From Ref. 8.

Table 1 Abbreviations and Their Meanings

CK (cytokeratin: pancytokeratin KL1, AE1/AE3
CK5/6, CK7, CK14, CK19, CK20)
CD45 (leucocyte common antigen)
S-100P (S-100 Protein)
EMA (epithelial membrane antigen)
CD20 (B lymphoid cell)
CD3 (T lymphoid cell)
CD10 (lymphoid precursor cell, some epithelial cells marker)
CD15 (granulocytes, Reed-Sternberg cell, adenocarcinoma marker)
CD30 (activation antigen)
ALK (anaplastic lymphoma kinase)
S-100 Protein, HMB45, Melan-A, PNL2 (melanocytic markers)
MSA (muscle specific actin)
DES (desmin, striated muscle)
CD31, CD34 (vascular marker)
CD68 (histiocytic marker)
CD99 (PNET marker)
CD117 (c-kit)
VIM (vimentin)
Calretinin, HBME1 (mesothelial markers)
BerEP4 (epithelial glycoprotein)
PLAP (placenta-like alkaline phosphatase)
AFP (α-Fetoprotein)
β-HCG (human chorionic gonadotropin)
CGA (chromogranin A)
SYN (synaptophysin)
NSE (neurone-specific enolase)
CEA (carcinoembryonic antigen)
CDX2 (intestinal transcription factor)
HepPar1 (hepatocytic antigen)
PSA (prostate-specific antigen)
TTF-1 (thyroid transcription factor-1)
GCDFP (gross cystic disease fluid protein)
ER (estrogene receptor)
PR (progesterone receptor)
GFAP (glial fibrillary acidic protein)
NF (neurofilament protein)
HER2 (c-erbB-2 oncoprotein)
EGFR (epidermal growth factor)
VEGF (vascular endothelial growth factor)

STRATEGIES FOR SPECIFIC HISTOPATHOLOGICAL TYPES

Undifferentiated Malignant Tumor

Immunohistochemistry could solve over 90% of cases presenting as undifferentiated malignant tumors by using a short panel of antibodies directed against epithelial antigens (panCK as AE1/AE3 or KL1), lymphoid antigen (CD45), and melanocytic antigen (S-100P) (Fig. 1).

Appropriate therapy and better prognostic entities justify using additional antibodies for difficult cases. For instance, lymphomas such as anaplastic large cell lymphoma (CD45−, EMA+, CD30+, ALK+) might present characteristics and an immunohistochemical phenotype that might lead to confusion with undifferentiated carcinoma. Some large B cell lymphomas (CD45+, CD20+, ...) or T cell lymphomas (CD45+, CD3+, ...) or Hodgkin's disease (EMA+, CD15+, CD30+, ...) might be difficult to discriminate as well.

It is noteworthy that diagnosis of extragonadal germ cell tumors, such as embryonal carcinoma (AFP+/−, CD30+) or yolk sac tumor (AFP+), choriocarcinoma (β-HCG+), and seminoma (PLAP+, VIM+, CD117+, focal CK+), is difficult to make on small samples and may require immunohistochemical data (12). S-100P, HMB45, and new antibodies as Melan-A/Mart1 and PNL2 have allowed improvements in the diagnosis of melanoma and its distinction from histological mimics (13,14).

Many markers have been identified for sarcomas (VIM, MSA, caldesmone, DES, myogenin, S-100P, CD31, CD34, CD68, CD117, ...). However, some sarcomas, such as synovial or epithelioid sarcoma, may coexpress epithelial (panCK) and mesenchymal (VIM) markers. Nevertheless, VIM is of limited interest because of its poor specificity. Malignant peripheral nerve sheath tumors and some liposarcomas express S-100P. PNET such as Ewing sarcomas express CD 99. It is unusual, however, to encounter this situation, except with small tumoral samples (15).

Once all these aforementioned and sometimes very chemosensitive entities (i.e., lymphoma, germ cell tumors) have been ruled out, the diagnosis of undifferentiated carcinoma is made. An algorithm is proposed to identify the exact histopathological type (Fig. 2). Despite the clinical and immunohistochemical data, diagnosis of undifferentiated malignant tumor will be retained in 10% of cases, without any reference to tumoral origin.

Undifferentiated Carcinoma or Adenocarcinoma (panCK+, CD45−, S-100P−)

Adenocarcinomas represent more than 50% of the CUP. In the diagnostic process of adenocarcinoma and undifferentiated carcinoma, despite their usual different morphology, the same algorithm can be used (Fig. 2). First, the neuroendocrine markers (CGA, SYN, CD56, CD57, NSE, ...) must be used to diagnose neuroendocrine tumors of an unknown primary site because these neoplasms may require a specific treatment. Thyrocalcitonin may help to identify metastasis from medullary carcinoma of the thyroid and should not be overlooked (16). In practice, the best recommended choice is to assess the reactivity of the CUP with two antibodies directed against CK7 and CK20, respectively (9,11,17,18). It is a well-known fact that the typical phenotype of poorly differentiated tumors can vary, but generally the unexpected positivity of CK7 or CK20 is weak and focal. If most tumors retain the CK7/CK20 phenotype during metastasis, the intratumoral heterogeneity remains the challenging problem. Finally, it is also mandatory to use additional antibodies, which are more or less specific, for different types of tumors. Four primary tumor sites are important, prostate, breast, ovary, and thyroid, for adequate treatment and better prognosis.

First Situation: Carcinoma CK7−/CK20−

Hepatocellular carcinomas (AFP with weak sensitivity) have a cytoplasmic expression of HepPar1, a CD34+ expression of sinusoids and a canalicular expression of CEA (polyclonal antibody), and CD10 (because of a cross-reaction with the biliary canalicular glycoprotein) (19–22). Most renal cell carcinomas (usually VIM+) express CD10 (23). Except rare cases, prostatic acid phosphatase and PSA are highly specific for prostatic carcinoma (7,11). Squamous cell carcinoma and most neuroendocrine carcinomas also share this phenotype CK7−/CK20− and express EMA.

Second Situation: Carcinoma CK7−/CK20+

The main neoplasm with this phenotype is colorectal carcinoma with occasionally a weak and focal expression of CK7 and usually CEA+ (nonspecific). CDX2 is an interesting but nonspecific new marker (24–26). Merkel cell carcinoma can be differentiated from cutaneous metastastic carcinoma using other antibodies (CGA, paranuclear focal dot-like panCK+, EMA+, NF+).

Third Situation: Carcinoma CK7+/CK20−

About 90% of lung adenocarcinomas share this phenotype. Moreover, 70% of primitive nonmucinous adenocarcinomas of the lung express TTF-1 (nuclear immunostaining) (27). Breast carcinomas express EMA, GCDFP, ER, PR, although poorly differentiated carcinomas might be negative for these markers. However, some extramammary carcinomas can express hormonal receptors. The situation is similar to the discriminative expression of CD10 (28) for endometrial and nonmucinous ovarian carcinomas. Thyroid carcinomas are generally strongly positive for thyroglobulin and TTF-1 but weakly positive in poorly differentiated carcinomas. Cholangiocellular carcinomas express CEA and CK19. However, differential diagnosis can be very difficult to make in liver metastasis of mucinous adenocarcinomas.

Fourth Situation: Carcinoma CK7+/CK20+

Pancreatic, gastric (CDX2+), and biliary carcinomas strongly express CEA. Mucinous ovarian (ER+, PR+, ...) as urothelial (uroplakin+, specific but weakly sensitive) carcinomas have this phenotype (29).

Squamous Cell (Epidermoid) Carcinoma

Routine hematoxylin–eosin allows the diagnosis of most cases but sometimes poorly differentiated squamous cell carcinoma can benefit from immunohistochemistry (CK5/6, CK14) (30,31).

STRATEGIES DEPENDING ON ANATOMIC LOCALIZATION

1. *Lymph node metastasis.* In CUP located in midline lymph nodes, lymphomas, and generally extragonadal germ cell tumors must be ruled out by appropriate immunostaining (see previous sections).
2. *Serous metastasis.* Malignant mesothelioma is sometimes difficult to differentiate from a metastatic pleural or peritoneal spread of lung carcinoma. The typical immunophenotype is: EMA+, calretinin+, CK5/6+, HBME1+, CD15 (LeuM1)−, BerEP4−, CEA−, ...), but "mesothelioma" markers can react with different subsets of lung carcinoma with a variable frequency (32). Peritoneal carcinomatosis should be distinguished from primary papillary serous peritoneal carcinoma and in young patients from desmoplastic round small cell tumor (CK+, DES+, ...).
3. *Liver metastasis.* Hepatocellular and cholangiocellular carcinomas have distinctive characteristic phenotypes. Liver metastasis from digestive adenocarcinoma can be difficult to rule out for a primary cholangiocellular carcinoma.
4. *Pulmonary metastasis.* Primary bronchial adenocarcinoma is sometimes difficult to diagnose on small samples.
5. *Brain metastasis.* An undifferentiated malignant tumor needs to be discriminated from a primary cerebral tumor (GFAP+).
6. *Bone metastasis.* Bone decalcification can destroy some antigens and particularly nuclear antigens. Unexpected reactivity, such as focal PSA or ER labeling for some lung tumors, must be kept in mind.
7. *Skin metastasis.* Merkel cell carcinoma (CGA+, CK20+, NF+, ...) and skin metastasis of undifferentiated carcinomas are sometimes difficult to tell apart.

TARGETED TREATMENT OF CUP

The development of a novel approach for targeted treatment of cancer, alone or combined with chemotherapy, often implies an immunohistopathological assessment. Such specific therapies may be investigated in CUP in the future. Several new antibodies directed against targets such as HER2 (c-erbB-2), CD117 (c-kit), EGFR, and VEGF are available for immunohistochemistry purpose. Some of these antibodies mark focally and weakly malignant tumors, whatever their histopathological type (33–37). Their assessment in CUPs is underway (38). Actually, our knowledge of how to best optimize such treatment is still unfolding.

CONCLUSION

Efficient management of CUP is closely related with a pluridisciplinar approach involving both the clinician and the pathologist. Such cooperative work entails a careful clinical history and a precise diagnostic investigation at the pathology level, based on tumor localization, morphology, and immunohistochemistry. This technique is a cost-effective tool that provides valuable clues for the clinician (1,39,40).

REFERENCES

1. Nissenblatt MJ. The CUP syndrome (carcinoma of unknown primary). Cancer Treat Rev 1981; 8:211–224.
2. Abbruzzese JL, Abbruzzese MC, Hess KR, Raber MN, Lenzi R, Frost P. Unknown primary carcinoma: natural history and prognostic factors in 657 consecutive patients. J Clin Oncol 1994; 12:1272–1280.
3. Lenzi R, Hess KR, Abbruzzese MC, Raber MN, Ordonez NG, Abbruzzese JL. Poorly differentiated carcinoma and poorly differentiated adenocarcinoma of unknown origin: favorable subsets of patients with unknown-primary carcinoma? J Clin Oncol 1997; 15:2056–2066.
4. Culine S, Lortholary A, Voigt JJ, et al. Cisplatin in combination with either Gemcitabine or Irinotecan in carcinomas of unknown primary site: results of a randomized phase II study-trial for the French Study Group on Carcinomas of Unknown Primary (GEFCAPI 01). J Clin Oncol 2003; 21:3479–3482.
5. De Young BR, Wick MR. Immunohistologic evaluation of metastatic carcinomas of unknown origin: an algorithmic approach. Semin Diagn Pathol 2000; 17:184–193.
6. Chan JKC. Advances in immunohistochemistry: impact on surgical pathology practice. Semin Diagn Pathol 2000; 17:170–177.
7. Dabbs DJ, ed. Carcinomatous differentiation and metastatic carcinoma of unknown primary. Diagnostic Immunohistochemistry. New York: Churchill Livingstone, 2002:163–196.
8. Bugat R, Bataillard A, Lesimple T, et al. Standards, options et recommandations 2002 pour la prise en charge des patients atteints de carcinome de site primitif inconnu (rapport intégral). FNCLCC. Montrouge: J Libbey Eurotext, 2004.
9. Bugat R, Bataillard A, Lesimple T, et al. Summary of the standards, options and recommendations for the management of patients with carcinoma of unknown primary site. Br J Cancer 2003; 89(suppl 1):59–66.

10. Lesimple T, Voigt JJ, Bataillard A, et al. Recommandations pour la pratique clinique: Standards, Options et Recommandations 2002 pour le diagnostic des carcinomes de site primitif inconnu. Bull Cancer 2003; 90:1071–1096.
11. Gown AM, Bacchi CE. Cost effective immunohistochemistry. 85th Annual Meeting. United States and Canadian Academy of Pathology. Washington, March, 1996.
12. Suster S, Moran CA, Dominguez-Malagon H, Quevedo-Blanco P. Germ cell tumors of the mediastinum and testis: a comparative immunohistochemical study of 120 cases. Hum Pathol 1998; 29:737–742.
13. Busam K. The use and application of special techniques in assessing melanocytic tumours. Pathology 2004; 36:462–469.
14. Rochaix P, Lacroix-Triki M, Lamant L, et al. PNL2, a new monoclonal antibody directed against a fixative-resistant melanocyte antigen. Mod Pathol 2003; 16:481–490.
15. Coindre JM. Immunohistochemistry in the diagnosis of soft tissue tumours. Histopathology 2003; 43:1–16.
16. Wick MR. Immunohistology of neuroendocrine and neuroectodermal tumors. Semin Diagn Pathol 2000; 17:194–203.
17. Tot T. Cytokeratins 20 and 7 as biomarkers: usefulness in discriminating primary from metastatic adenocarcinoma. Eur J Cancer 2002; 38:758–763.
18. Kende AI, Carr NJ, Sobin LH. Expression of cytokeratins 7 and 20 in carcinomas of the gastrointestinal tract. Histopathology 2003; 42:137–140.
19. Chu PG, Ishizawa S, Wu E, Weiss LM. Hepatocyte antigen as a marker of hepatocellular carcinoma. An immunohistochemical comparison to carcinoembryonic antigen, CD10, and Alpha-Fetoprotein. Am J Surg Pathol 2002; 26: 978–988.
20. Borscheri N, Roessner A, Rocken C. Canalicular immunostaining of neprilysin (CD10) as a diagnostic marker for hepatocellular carcinomas. Am J Surg Pathol 2001; 25:1297–1303.
21. Tickoo SK, Zee SY, Obiekwe S, et al. Combined hepatocellular-cholangiocarcinoma. A histopathologic, immunohistochemical, and in situ hybridization study. Am J Surg Pathol 2002; 26:989–997.
22. Terracciano LM, Glatz K, Mhawech P, et al. Hepatoid adenocarcinoma with liver metastasis mimicking hepatocellular carcinoma. An immunohistochemical and molecular study of eight cases. Am J Surg Pathol 2003; 27:1302–1312.
23. Avery AK, Beckstead J, Renshaw A, Corless CL. Use of antibodies to RCC and CD10 in the differential diagnosis of renal neoplasms. Am J Surg Pathol 2000; 24:203–210.
24. Barbareschi M, Murer B, Colby TV, et al. CDX-2 homeobox gene expression is a reliable marker of colorectal adenocarcinoma metastases to the lungs. Am J Surg Pathol 2003; 27:141–149.
25. Werling RW, Yaziji H, Bacchi CE, Gown AM. CDX-2, a highly sensitive and specific marker of adenocarcinomas of intestinal origin. An immunohistochemical survey of 476 primary and metastatic carcinomas. Am J Surg Pathol 2003; 27:303–310.
26. Li MK, Folpe AL. CDX-2, a new marker for adenocarcinoma of gastrointestinal origin. Adv Anat Pathol 2004; 11:101–105.

27. Yatabe Y, Mitsudomi T, Takahashi T. TTF-1 expression in pulmonary adenocarcinomas. Am J Surg Pathol 2002; 26:767–773.
28. Ordi J, Romagosa C, Tavassoli FA, et al. CD10 expression in epithelial tissues and tumors of the gynecologic tract. A useful marker in the diagnosis of mesonephric, trophoblastic and clear cell tumors. Am J Surg Pathol 2003; 27:178–186.
29. Parker DC, Folpe AL, Bell J, et al. Potential utility of uroplakin III, thrombomodulin, high molecular weight cytokeratin, and cytokeratin 20 in noninvasive, invasive and metastatic urothelial (transitional cell) carcinomas. Am J Surg Pathol 2003; 27:1–10.
30. Nieder C, Ang KK. Cervical lymph node metastases from occult squamous cell carcinoma. Curr Treat Options Oncol 2002; 3:33–40.
31. Chu PG, Lyda MH, Weiss LM. Cytokeratin 14 expression in epithelial neoplasms: a survey of 435 cases with emphasis on its value in differentiating squamous cell carcinomas from other epithelial tumours. Histopathology 2001; 39:9–16.
32. Miettinen M, Sarlomo-Rikala M. Expression of calretinin, thrombomodulin, keratin 5, and mesothelin in lung carcinomas of different types. An immunohistochemical analysis of 596 tumors in comparison with epithelioid mesotheliomas of the pleura. Am J Surg Pathol 2003; 27:150–158.
33. Baselga J. New therapeutic agents targeting the epidermal growth factor. J Clin Oncol 2000; 18:54–59.
34. Hainsworth JD, Lennington WJ, Greco FA. Overexpression of Her-2 in patients with poorly differentiated carcinoma or poorly differentiated adenocarcinoma of unknown primary site. J Clin Oncol 2000; 18:623–635.
35. Voigt JJ, Culine S, Le SimpleT, et al. Carcinomes de site primitif inconnu. HER-2, EGFR et c-kit sont-ils de nouvelles cibles thérapeutiques? Ann Pathol 2003; 23(suppl 1):126.
36. Mosesson Y, Yarden Y. Oncogenic growth factor receptors: implications for signal transduction therapy. Semin Cancer Biol 2004; 14:262–270.
37. Le Guen Y, Sabatier L, Le Chevalier T, Soria JC. Thérapeutiques moléculaires ciblées en cancérologie bronchique. Bull Cancer 2003; 90:1055–1061.
38. Fizazi K, Voigt JJ, Lesimple T, et al. Carcinoma of unknown primary (CUP): are tyrosine kinase receptors HER-2, EGF-R, and c-kit suitable targets for therapy? Proc Am Soc Clin Oncol 2003; 22:883.
39. Pavlidis N, Briasoulis E, Hainsworth J, Greco FA. Diagnostic and therapeutic management of cancer of an unknown primary. Eur J Cancer 2003; 39: 1990–2005.
40. Coindre JM, Blanc-Vincent MP, Collin F, Mac Grogan G, Balaton A, Voigt JJ. Standards, options et recommandations: conduite à tenir devant une lésion de diagnostic anatomo-cytopathologique difficile en cancérologie. Ann Pathol 2003; 23:460–470.

4

The Importance of Identifying CUP Subsets

Nicholas Pavlidis

*Department of Medical Oncology, Ioannina University Hospital,
Ioannina, Greece*

Yacine Merrouche

Institut de Cancérologie de la Loire, Saint Priest en Jarez, France

INTRODUCTION

Cancer of unknown primary (CUP) origin is the seventh to eighth most frequent malignancy and the fourth commonest cause of cancer death. It accounts for 3% to 5% of all malignant neoplasms (1–3).

CUP is defined as a histologically confirmed diagnosis of malignancy in patients with unremarkable medical history and physical examination, with normal routine blood tests, urine and stool tests, noncontributory immuno-histochemical investigation as well as normal chest X ray, abdominal and pelvic computed tomography (CT), or mammography in certain cases (4–6).

Median age at diagnosis is approximately 60 years with male pre-dilection. The natural history of CUP consists of an early metastatic dissemination, clinical absence of primary site, aggressive behavior, and an unpredictable metastatic pattern (7). Research on biological or molecular mechanisms of CUP is still limited. Results of oncogene overexpression remain controversial (6).

The diagnostic investigation to identify the primary tumor should always follow certain algorithms in order to avoid time and money consumption (6,8). Despite thorough diagnostic work-up using modern pathological and imaging procedures, the frequency of antemortem detection of primary tumor is still around 20% of the cases (7,9–19).

CUP does not represent a single disease but on the contrary it does include more than one clinicopathological entities. In this chapter we intend to describe the clinical picture, natural history, and differential diagnosis of all known clinicopathological entities of patients with CUP.

HISTOPATHOLOGICAL SUBTYPES

Patients with CUP are classified into four major subtypes by routine light microscopy diagnosis:

1. *Adenocarcinomas.* Fifty percent of CUP patients will be diagnosed with well to moderately differentiated metastatic adenocarcinoma.
2. *Poorly or undifferentiated carcinomas.* Almost 30% of cases will carry the diagnosis of poorly or undifferentiated carcinoma.
3. *Squamous cell carcinomas.* This subtype represents the 15% of all CUP patients.
4. *Undifferentiated neoplasms.* Five percent will be diagnosed as undifferentiated neoplasms, most of which will be further characterized by modern immunohistopathology as neuroendocrine tumors, lymphomas, germ cell tumors, melanomas, or sarcomas (Table 1) (6,20).

Table 1 Histopathological Subtypes of CUP

Subtypes	Incidence (%)
Adenocarcinoma	
Well to moderately differentiated	50
Poorly or undifferentiated	30
Squamous cell carcinoma	15
Undifferentiated neoplasms	5
Not specified carcinoma	
Neuroendocrine tumors	
Lymphomas	
Germ cell tumors	
Melanomas	
Sarcomas	
Embryonal malignances	

Abbreviation: CUP, cancer of unknown primary site.

CLINICOPATHOLOGICAL ENTITIES

CUP subsets differ in terms of histopathological and clinical features. The characterization of a certain clinicopathological entity is based on various clinical or nonclinical parameters such as age, sex, histopathology, clinical presentation, and organ or site involvement (Table 2).

Proper differential diagnosis and recognition of CUP clinicopathological subsets will provide an enormous help to the clinician for a precise diagnostic investigation and for an appropriate therapeutic management.

Several subsets will have a better response to systemic or local treatment and will follow a more favorable prognosis. Satisfactory local control

Table 2 Distinct Clinicopathological Entities of Patients with CUP

Site of involvement	Histopathology
Liver (mainly) *and/or other organs*	Adenocarcinoma (moderately or poorly differentiated)
Lymph nodes	
Mediastinal–retroperitoneal (midline distribution)	Undifferentiated or poorly differentiated carcinoma
Axillary	Adenocarcinoma (well to poorly differentiated)
Cervical	Squamous cell carcinoma
Inguinal	Undifferentiated carcinoma, squamous, mixed squamous/adenocarcinoma
Peritoneal cavity	
Peritoneal adenocarcinomatosis in females	Papillary or serous adenocarcinoma ($\pm$ psammoma bodies)
Malignant ascites of other unknown origin	Mucin–producing adenocarcinoma (moderately or poorly differentiated $\pm$ signet ring cells)
Lungs	
Pulmonary metastases	Adenocarcinoma (various differentiation)
Pleural effusions	Adenocarcinoma (moderately or poorly differentiated)
Bones (solitary or multiple)	Adenocarcinoma (various differentiation)
Brain (solitary or multiple)	Adenocarcinoma (various differentiations or squamous cell carcinoma)
Neuroendocrine tumors	Poorly differentiated carcinoma with neuroendocrine features (mainly), low-grade neuroendocrine carcinomas, small cell anaplastic carcinomas
Malignant melanoma	Undifferentiated neoplasm with melanoma features

Abbreviation: CUP, cancer of unknown primary site.

or long survivors can be observed. However, other subsets are not chemo-sensitive and have short survival rates.

FAVORABLE SUBSETS (TABLE 3)

Metastatic Disease to the Lymph Nodes

Subset of Nodal Midline Distribution
(Mediastinal–Retroperitoneal Involvement)

In this group of patients the mediastinal and retroperitoneal lymph nodes are predominantly involved. The supraclavicular and cervical nodes as well as the lungs are less frequently affected. This subset was first described in 1979 as an "extragonadal germ cell syndrome." Today, it is characterized as an undifferentiated or poorly differentiated carcinoma of midline distribution.

It is more common in males of approximately 50 years and is a rapidly progressive disease. In 25% of these cases, molecular genetic analysis shows an abnormality of isochromosome of the short arm of chromosome 12i (12p) or a deletion in 12p.

In addition, serum human chorionic gonadotropin (β-HCG) or α-fetoprotein (AFP) are elevated in around 20% of the cases. This subset is responsive to platinum-based chemotherapy with almost 50% response rates and 15% long-term survivors (21–27).

Currow et al. observed a negative association between elevated serum β-HCG and AFP markers and response to cisplatin-based chemotherapy in CUP patients. However, it seems that the reported patients do not belong to the known subset of nodal midline distribution patients (28).

Subset of Isolated Metastases to Axillary Nodes

This is mainly a female disease and resembles stage II or III breast cancer patients, although only 0.3% of these patients will be eventually diagnosed

Table 3 Favorable Subsets of CUP

Poorly differentiated carcinoma with midline distribution
   (extragonadal germ cell syndrome)
Women with papillary adenocarcinoma of peritoneal cavity
Women with adenocarcinoma involving only axillary lymph nodes
Squamous cell carcinoma involving cervical lymph nodes
Isolated inguinal adenopathy (squamous cell carcinoma)
Poorly differentiated neuroendocrine carcinomas
Men with blastic bone metastases and elevated PSA (adenocarcinoma)
Patients with a single, small, potentially resectable tumor

Abbreviations: CUP, cancer of unknown primary site; PSA, prostate specific antigen.

with breast carcinoma. The median age is 52 years ranging from 20 to 80 years. Biopsy is usually compatible with an invasive ductal adenocarcinoma of grade III, while estrogen and progesterone receptors are positive in 20% to 30% of the cases. Mammography and/or ultrasound of the breast is an important diagnostic investigation. A breast magnetic resonance could be useful after a negative mammography. At diagnosis, 70% of the patients have N_1 disease and very rarely—in less than 5%—metastatic sites can be discovered. Males are very rarely affected by this subset and they carry a worse prognosis. The therapeutic management should be similar to females with stage II to III breast cancer (29–32).

Subset of Cervical or Supraclavicular Nodal Involvement with Squamous Histology

Patients presented with metastatic squamous cell carcinoma of the upper or middle cervical lymph node; a primary head and neck tumor should always be suspected. However, in patients with lower or subclavicular nodal metastases, lungs are the most possible hidden primary sites. Cervical nodal metastases from clinically undetectable primary squamous cell carcinoma accounts for 1% to 2% of head–neck malignancies, although approximately 30% of them will subsequently have a primary tumor detected during the clinical course of the disease.

Extensive endoscopic evaluation of the head–neck area and lungs as well as facial and neck CT scans are recommended. 18-F-Fluorodeoxyglucose (FDG)-position emission tomography (PET) has shown adequate sensitivity in detecting primary sites. Serology for Epstein–Barr virus or detection of DNA by in situ hybridization could be performed for diagnosis of an undifferentiated nasopharyngeal carcinoma, particularly for young male patient native from North Africa or South East Asia.

Patients with upper or middle cervical lymph node involvement from a squamous type carcinoma should be treated as locally advanced head and neck cancer patients. Relatively good responses and satisfactory five-year survival rates can be seen (33,34).

Subset of Inguinal Nodal Involvement

This is a quite rare subset of either undifferentiated or squamous histology. Primary tumors in the genital or anorectal areas should always be ruled out. An extensive clinical examination of vulva, vagina, cervix, penis, and scrotum should be performed. A differential diagnosis from a lymphoma or an amelanotic melanoma of unknown primary site should also be considered (35,36).

Peritoneal Papillary Serous Carcinomatosis in Women

Initially, this entity has been reported in 1959, but it was characterized as a separated CUP subset almost 20 years later. Today, peritoneal serous papillary carcinoma is a recognized distinct clinicopathological entity in which peritoneal carcinomatosis of ovarian serous type is found in the abdomen and/or pelvis.

These patients are presented with ascites and peritoneal masses without detection of a primary tumor in the ovaries on exploratory laparotomy. Metastases outside the peritoneal cavity are unusual. The median age is 60 years. Most patients have elevated serum levels of CA 125. Very few cases of primary papillary serous carcinoma of the peritoneum have been reported in men (37,38).

In clinical practice, female peritoneal papillary serous carcinomatosis should be differentiated from peritoneal mesothelioma, pseudomyxoma peritonii, and malignant ascites arising from other systems.

Optimal therapeutic management of these women is similar to stage III ovarian cancer and includes surgical cytoreduction followed by platinum-based chemotherapy. Favorable responses are commonly seen (39–41).

Metastatic Neuroendocrine Carcinomas

Neuroendocrine malignant tumors represent a broad spectrum of neoplasms most of which have a known primary site. Histopathologically, three distinct subtypes have been recognized: (i) the low-grade neuroendocrine carcinomas, i.e., carcinoids or islet-cell tumors, (ii) the small cell anaplastic pulmonary or extrapulmonary carcinoma, and (iii) the poorly differentiated carcinoma or adenocarcinoma of an unknown primary origin with neuroendocrine features. These three subsets reflect also distinct clinicopathological entities.

The latter clinicopathological entity belongs to the favorable subsets of CUP and affects more commonly males. It involves predominantly lymph nodes and some patients share common features with the poorly differentiated carcinoma of nodal midline distribution. Other splachnic organs can also be the dominant metastatic sites. Immunohistochemically, they express positive immunoperoxidase staining for chromogranin, synaptophysin, or neuron-specific enolase.

These tumors are treated with platinum-containing combination chemotherapy. Considerable responses including complete remissions and prolonged survival have been observed (20,27,42).

Osteoblastic Bone Metastases with Elevated PSA in Men

This rare subset includes male patients presented with mainly metastatic bone disease of osteoblastic type and an increased serum prostate specific antigen (PSA). The biopsy shows an adenocarcinoma of various differentiation. Immunoperoxidase staining with PSA should always be requested. The bone metastatic lesions could be either solitary or multiple. The recommended treatment is hormonal manipulation similar to the management of prostate cancer (20,43,44).

Patients with a Single Metastatic Site

This is also a rare entity where patients are presented with a single site of metastasis. The metastatic sites could be either a single lymph node, i.e., cervical, supraclavicular, or inguinal, or a single metastatic site in the liver, brain, lungs, or elsewhere. All patients should be subjected to surgical removal of the single metastatic lesion followed by local radiotherapy. In cases of poorly differentiated carcinomas adjuvant chemotherapy should also be considered (6).

UNFAVORABLE SUBSETS (TABLE 4)

Unfortunately, the unfavorable group of CUP is the most common diagnosis among these patients. Most of them present with multiple metastatic sites of well to poorly differentiated adenocarcinoma and generally they have poor response to chemotherapy and short median survival.

Metastatic Adenocarcinoma to the Liver and/or to Multiple Other Sites

This subset comprises the most common diagnosis of CUP accounting for more than one-fourth of the cases. The median age of these patients is higher than those with favorable CUP subsets approaching the seventh decade of life. Multiple liver metastatic lesions is the main clinical finding, although other metastatic sites to other organs are also common at the time of diagnosis. Metastatic adenocarcinoma of various differentiations is the usual histological diagnosis. Immunohistochemical staining with neuroendocrine markers should always be requested.

In the majority of the cases extensive radiological or endoscopic investigations fail to detect the primary site. Coloscopy could be useful in the presence of exclusive respectable liver metastases. Epithelial serum tumor markers could be elevated but had no prognostic or predictive value. The prognosis of these patients is poor with a median survival of six to nine months (8,20,45–47).

Table 4 Unfavorable Subsets of CUP

Adenocarcinoma metastatic to the liver or other organs
Nonpapillary malignant ascites (adenocarcinoma)
Multiple cerebral metastases (adeno or squamous carcinoma)
Multiple lung/pleural metastases (adenocarcinoma)
Multiple metastatic bone disease (adenocarcinoma)

Abbreviation: CUP, cancer of unknown primary site.

It is worthwhile to address that in all studies evaluating prognostic factors in patients with CUP, liver metastases along with performance status and serum LDH were found to be the most adverse prognostic variables (48–50).

Metastatic CUP to the Lungs

Patients with Only Parenchymal Metastases

These patients present with symptoms and signs attributed to the lung lesions. Radiological examinations reveal exclusively pulmonary paranechymal disease, while bronchoscopy fails to identify the primary tumor. Histological diagnosis is compatible with adenocarcinoma. The prognosis of most of these patients is dismal. In cases of young male patients, extragonadal metastatic disease should be ruled out (6,8,20,45).

Patients with Isolated Malignant Pleural Effusion

Although pleural involvement is a common finding in primary malignancies and in CUP patients, an isolated manifestation without a known primary is found in only 7%. Histologically, an adenocarcinoma is usually diagnosed. In women a breast or ovarian cancer should be excluded, while in men with smoking history lung cancer or mesothelioma should be included in the differential diagnosis. In general, the prognosis of this CUP entity has a poor prognosis (6,8,20).

Peritoneal Carcinomatosis from Nongynecologic Malignancies

Males or females could be presented with malignant ascites from a nonpapillary serous adenocarcinoma of unknown primary site. In patients with a mucin-producing adenocarcinoma with or without signet ring cells, a gastrointestinal malignancy should be suspected. The median age of this subset is around 67 years and is presented with stage III and IV peritoneal carcinomatosis according to Gilly's staging classification. Overall median survival is only 1.5 month with very poor response to chemotherapy (51).

Multiple Cerebral Metastases

In contrast to the single brain metastatic subset, the subgroup of CUP patients with multiple cerebral metastases carries a poor prognosis. In almost 15% of all patients with CNS metastases no primary tumor can be detected elsewhere. Patients are presented with a variety of neurological symptoms and signs. Biopsy of an intracranial lesion usually reveals a metastatic adenocarcinoma or a squamous cell carcinoma (52–54).

Multiple Metastatic Bone Disease

Bone metastases is a frequent manifestation in CUP patients. However, exclusive bone metastatic lesions are not a very common subset. These patients present with a clinical picture attributed to osseous metastatic sites, i.e., bone pain or fracture. Histologically, adenocarcinoma is the usual diagnosis. In men prostatic cancer and in women breast cancer should always be ruled out. Even if primary diagnosis in these patients cannot be made, starting treatment with an endocrine manipulation may be considered. Generally, the outcome remains poor (43,44).

REFERENCES

1. Ries LAG, Eisner MP, Kosary CL, et al. SEER Cancer Statistics Review. National Cancer Institute, 1999.
2. Levi F, Te VC, Erler G, Randimbison L, La Vecchia C. Epidemiology of unknown primary tumors. Eur J Cancer 2002; 38:1810–1812.
3. Van de Wouw AJ, Janssen-Heijnen MLG, Coebergh JWW, Hillen HF. Epidemiology of unknown primary tumors; incidence and population-based survival of 1285 patients in Southeast Netherlands, 1984–1992. Eur J Cancer 2002; 38:409–413.
4. Frost P, Raber MN, Abbruzzese JL. Unknown primary tumors as a unique clinical and biologic entity: a hypothesis. Cancer Bull 1989; 41:139–141.
5. Abbruzzese JL, Abbruzzese MC, Lenzi R, Hess KR, Raber MN. Analysis of a diagnostic strategy for patients with suspected tumors of unknown origin. J Clin Oncol 1995; 13:2094–2103.
6. Pavlidis N, Briasoulis E, Hainsworth J, Greco FA. Diagnostic and therapeutic management of cancer of an unknown primary. Eur J Cancer 2003; 39: 1990–2005.
7. Nystrom JS, Weiner JM, Hellelfinger-Juttner J, Irwin LE, Bateman JR, Wolf RM. Metastatic and histologic presentation in unknown primary cancer. Semin Oncol 1977; 4:53–58.
8. Bugat R, Bataillard A, Lesimple T, et al. Summary of the standards, options and recommendations for the management of patients with carcinoma of unknown primary site. Br J Cancer 2003; 89(suppl 1):S59–S66.
9. Holmes FF, Fouts TL. Metastatic cancer of unknown primary site. Cancer 1970; 26:816–820.
10. Stewart J, Tattersall M, Woods R, Fox R. Unknown primary adenocarcinoma: incidence of overinvestigation and natural history. Br Med J 1979; 1:1530–1533.
11. Smith P, Krementz E, Chapman W. Metastatic cancer without a detectable primary site. Am J Surg 1967; 113:633–637.
12. Probert J. Secondary carcinoma in cervical lymph nodes with an occult primary tumor. A review of 61 patients including their response to radiotherapy. Clin Radiol 1970; 21:211–218.
13. Pico J, Frias Z, Bosch A. Cervical lymph node metastases from carcinoma of undetermined origin. Am J Roentgenol 1971; 111:95–102.
14. Lleander V, Goldstein G, Horsley J. Chemotherapy in the management of metastatic cancer of unknown primary site. Oncology 1972; 26:265–270.
15. Moertel C, Reitemeier R, Schutt A, et al. Treatment of the patient with adenocarcinoma of unknown origin. Cancer 1972; 30:1469–1472.
16. Didolkar M, Fanous N, Elias E, et al. Metastatic carcinomas from occult primary tumors. A study of 254 patients. Ann Surg 1977; 186:625–630.

17. Snyder R, Mavligit G, Valdivieso M. Adenocarcinoma of unknown primary site: a clinicopathological study. Med Pediatr Oncol 1979; 6:289–294.
18. Steckel R, Kagan R. Diagnostic persistence in working-up metastatic cancer with an unknown primary site. Radiology 1980; 134:367–369.
19. Shildt R, Kennedy P, Chen T, et al. Management of patients with metastatic adenocarcinoma of unknown origin: a Southwest Oncology Group Study. Cancer Treat Rep 1983; 67:77–79.
20. Greco FA, Hainsworth JD. Cancer of unknown primary site. In: DeVita TV, Hellman S, Rosenberg SA, eds. Cancer: Principles and Practice of Oncology. 4th ed. 1997:2423–2443.
21. Richardson RL, Greco FA, Wolff S, et al. Extragonadal germ cell malignancy: value of tumor markers in metastatic carcinoma in young men. Proc Am Soc Clin Oncol 1979; 20:204.
22. Fox RM, Woods RL, Tattersall MHN, McGovern VJ. Undifferentiated carcinoma in young men: the atypical teratoma syndrome. Lancet 1979; I: 1316–1318.
23. Richardson RL, Schoumacher R, Oldham RK, et al. The unrecognized extra-gonadal germ cell syndrome. Ann Intern Med 1981; 94:181–189.
24. Greco FA, Vaughn WK, Hainsworth JD. Advanced poorly differentiated carcinoma of unknown primary site: recognition of a treatable syndrome. Ann Intern Med 1986; 142:547–553.
25. Hainsworth JD, Wright EP, Gray GF, Greco FA. Poorly differentiated carcinoma of unknown primary site: correlation of light microscopic findings with response to cisplatin-based combination chemotherapy. J Clin Oncol 1987; 5:1275–1280.
26. Hainsworth JD, Johnson DH, Greco FA. Poorly differentiated neuroendocrine carcinoma of unknown primary site: a newly recognized clinicopathologic entity. Ann Intern Med 1988; 109:364–371.
27. Van der Gaast A, Verweij J, Henzen-Logmans SC, et al. Carcinoma of unknown primary: identification of a treatable subset. Ann Oncol 1990; 1:119–122.
28. Currow DC, Findlay M, Cox K, Harnett PR. Elevated germ cell markers in carcinoma of uncertain primary site do not predict response to platinum based chemotherapy. Eur J Cancer 1996; 32A:2357–2359.
29. Ellerbroek N, Holmes F, Singletary E, Evans H, Oswald M, Mc Neese M. Treatment of patients with isolated axillary nodal metastases from an occult primary carcinoma consistent with breast origin. Cancer 1990; 66:1461–1467.
30. Foroudi F, Tiver KW. Occult breast carcinoma presenting as axillary metastases. Int J Radiat Oncol Biol Phys 2000; 47:143–147.
31. Vlastos G, Jean ME, Mizza AN, et al. Feasibility of breast presentation in the treatment of occult primary carcinoma presenting with axillary metastases. Ann Surg Oncol 2001; 8:425–431.
32. Jackson B, Scott-Conner C, Moulder J. Axillary metastases from occult breast carcinoma: diagnosis and management. Am Surg 1995; 61:431–434.
33. Grau C, Johansen LV, Jakobsen J, Geertsen P, Andersen E, Jensen BB. Cervical lymph node metastases from unknown primary tumors. Results from a national survey by the Danish Society for Head and Neck Oncology. Radiother Oncol 2000; 55:121–129.

34. Nieder C, Gregoire V, Ang KK. Cervical lymph node metastases from occult squamous cell carcinoma: cut down a tree to get an apple? Int J Radiat Oncol Biol Phys 2001; 50:727–733.
35. Guarischi A, Keane TJ, Elhakim T. Metastatic inguinal nodes from an unknown primary neoplasm. A review of 56 cases. Cancer 1987; 19:572–577.
36. Casciato DA, Tabbarah HJ. Metastases of unknown origin. In: Haskell CM, ed. Cancer Treatment. 3rd ed. WB Saunders, 1990:798–814.
37. Shmueli E, Leider–Trejo L, Schwartz I, Aderka D, Inbar M. Primary papillary serous carcinoma of the peritoneum in a man. Ann Oncol 2001; 12:563–567.
38. Shah AI, Jayram L, Gani OS, et al. Papillary serous carcinoma of the peritoneum in a man: a case report. Cancer 1998; 82(5):860–866.
39. Chen KT, Flam MS. Peritoneal papillary serous carcinoma with long-term survival. Cancer 1986; 58:1371–1373.
40. Dalrymple JC, Bannatyne P, Russel P, et al. Extraovarian peritoneal serous papillary carcinoma. A clinicopathologic study of 31 cases. Cancer 1989; 64:110–115.
41. Ransom DT, Patel SR, Keeney GL, Malkasian GD, Edmonson JH. Papillary serous carcinoma of the peritoneum. Cancer 1990; 66:1091–1094.
42. Moertel CG, Kvols LK, O' Connell MJ, Rubin J. Treatment of neuroendocrine carcinomas with combined etoposide and cisplatin: evidence of major therapeutic activity in the anaplastic variants of these neoplasms. Cancer 1991; 68:227–233.
43. Tell DT, Khoury JM, Taylor HG, Veasey SP. Atypical metastasis from prostate cancer: clinical utility of the immunoperoxidase technique for prostate specific antigen. JAMA 1985; 253:3574–3579.
44. Gentile PS, Carloss HW, Huang TY, Yam LT, Lam WK. Disseminated prostatic carcinoma simulating primary lung cancer. Cancer 1988; 62:711–714.
45. Abbruzzese JL, Abbruzzese MC, Hess KR, Raber MN, Lenzi R, Frost P. Unknown primary carcinoma: natural history and prognostic factors in 657 consecutive patients. J Clin Oncol 1994; 12:1272–1280.
46. Ayoub JP, Hess KR, Abbruzzese MC, Lenzi R, Raber MN, Abbruzzese JC. Unknown primary tumors metastatic to liver. J Clin Oncol 1998; 16:2105–2112.
47. Hainsworth JD, Johnson DH, Greco FA. Cisplatin-based combination chemotherapy in the treatment of poorly differentiated carcinoma and poorly differentiated adenocarcinoma of unknown primary site: results of a 12-year experience. J Clin Oncol 1992; 10:912–922.
48. Kambhu SA, Kelsen DP, Fiore J, et al. Metastatic adenocarcinomas of unknown primary site: prognostic variables and treatment results. Am J Clin Oncol 1990; 13:55–60.
49. Van der Gaast A, Verweij J, Planting AST, et al. Simple prognostic model to predict survival in patients with undifferentiated carcinoma of unknown primary site. J Clin Oncol 1995; 13:1720–1725.
50. Culine S, Kramar A, Saghatchian M, et al. Development and validation of a prognostic model to predict the length of survival in patients with carcinomas of an unknown primary site. J Clin Oncol 2002; 20:4679–4683.
51. Sadeghi B, Arvieux C, Glehen D, et al. Peritoneal carcinomatosis from non-gynecologic malignancies. Results of the EVOCAPE 1 multicentric prospective study. Cancer 2000; 88:358–363.

52. Le Chevalier T, Smith FP, Caille P, Costans JP, Rouesse JG. Sites of primary malignancies in patients presenting with cerebral metastases. A review of 120 cases. Cancer 1985; 56:880–882.
53. Nguyen LN, Maor MH, Oswald MJ. Brain metastases as the only manifestation of an undetected primary tumor. Cancer 1998; 83:2181–2184.
54. Wen PY, Loeffler JS. Management of brain metastases. Oncology 1999; 13: 941–954.

5

Role of Positron Emission Tomography with 18F-Fluorodesoxyglucose (PET-FDG) in the Care of Carcinomas of an Unknown Primary Site

Etienne Garin

Nuclear Medicine Department, Eugene Marquis Centre, Rennes, France

Dirk Rades

Department of Radiation Oncology, University Medical Center Hamburg–Eppendorf, Hamburg, Germany

INTRODUCTION

Positron emission tomography with 18F-fluorodesoxyglucose (PET-FDG) could be used for the detection of the primary in cases of patient with carcinoma of an unknown primary site (CUP) and has been widely evaluated in this area. The most intensively explored situation is the form of cancer in patients presenting with cervical metastases of unknown primary. In such a situation, PET-FDG makes it possible to locate a primary in 33% of the patients and leads to a therapeutic modification for 35% of the patients. This examination should be carried out before the upper endoscopy, thus guiding the biopsies if possible. PET-FDG has been very little explored for patients presenting with metastases that are not cervical. On the basis of the small amount of data available, PET-FDG in this indication appears to localize the primary in 53% of cases, with an impact on the therapeutic care for 35% of the patients.

These results should be confirmed with large prospectives studies, in particular for patients with metastases other than cervical, because of the small number of published studies involving a small number of patients.

PET-FDG imagery depends on the detection of tumor tissues exhibiting a hyperconsumption of glucose (1). This phenomenon is related to an increase in aerobic glycolysis (1) that, amongst other things, is secondary to an increase in the glucose transporters (2). FDG is a glucose analog labeled with fluorine-18, which enters the cells by the same transport mechanism. Being also a substrate of hexokinase, it is phosphorylated on the 6 carbon position. On the other hand, FDG-6-phosphate is poorly metabolized by tumor cells and thus accumulates within them (3). PET-FDG has been used over the past 10 years in other countries in many pathologies (lung cancer, breast cancer, lymphomas, melanomas, cancers of ear–nose–throat, digestive system, etc.) (3,4). This functional and noninvasive imagery technique allows an exploration of the whole body during the same examination. In oncology, this usually concerns an area from the base of the cranium to the lesser pelvis. Faced with a tumor, the functional character of PET-FDG makes it possible to make a distinction between malignant lesions and other pathologies (benign tumors, inflammatory processes, etc.). This technique also enables the detection of tumor lesions of small size considered as nonsignificant with conventional imagery examinations.

As early as 1994, Rege et al. evoked the possibility of using PET-FDG to identify primaries among patients presenting with cervical metastases (5). Indeed, PET-FDG made it possible to locate a primary in two patients out of four who had cervical metastases of unknown primary, whereas the MRI was negative. Since then, a score of studies have been published as original articles targeted on the evaluation of PET-FDG in CUP. The majority of these studies are focused on the identification of the primary when confronted with cervical lymph-node metastases. Some of the studies, on the contrary, are not targeted and comprise varied presentations of CUP.

The prognosis of CUP patients depends on the stage of disease. Median survival is about 20 months for localized disease (lymph-node manifestation in one region only or one solitary visceral metastasis only) and about 7 months for disseminated disease (disseminated lymph node and/or visceral manifestation). The five-year survival rates are 30% to 35% and about 5%, respectively. The comparably good prognosis in case of localized disease offers an option for locally curative treatment. Thus, detection of the primary tumor and accurate staging are very important in order to select an appropriate risk adapted individual treatment concept. Because the prognosis for disseminated disease is poor, early detection of dissemination is important to avoid further diagnostic procedures that might be associated with discomfort for the patient.

PET-FDG AND CERVICAL METASTASES OF
UNKNOWN PRIMARY

Table 1 summarizes the diagnostic performances of PET-FDG in this targeted indication. PET-FDG is carried out with the aim of locating the primary tumor, in order to adapt, if possible, the best possible therapeutic approach. In this situation, the percentage identification of the primary varies from 7% to 60% according to different studies (6–19). By collecting together the results of the 14 studies targeted on this presentation of the CUP (6–18), the overall percentage of identification of the primary is 33%, corresponding to 102 cases out of 306. In addition, it is noteworthy that PET-FDG is highly sensitive in identifying the primary, with a success rate of 50% to 100% according to different studies. This point is important to stress, because it implies that if PET-FDG fails to identify the primary, there will then be very little chance of ever discovering it, even with long-term monitoring of the patients. Indeed, in cases where PET-FDG could not locate the primary, it was never detected later for 5 patients out of 5 in the study of Aassar et al. (9), 8 patients out of 9 in Braams et al. (7), 9 patients out of 10 in Safa et al. (12), and 18 patients out of 20 in Jungehülsing et al. (13). When the primary is discovered, it is generally localized at the level of the head and neck (Fig. 1) (6–10,13,15,18). However, one study reports a significant number of pulmonary primaries (14). In this study, out of fifteen detected primaries, seven were localized in the lungs (in six cases out of seven, the metastases corresponded to epidermoid carcinoma).

The absence of a thoracic computed axial tomography (CT) may partly explain these results (but this information is usually not available in the other studies either), while, in certain studies, the PET-FDG did not include the thorax or the totality of the thorax (8,9,11). On the other hand, the specificity of PET-FDG is a little lower than its sensitivity, given as 25% to 100% according to different studies, in particular due to false positives related to the presence of physiological uptake sites in the head and neck area (muscular uptakes in general) that are not always identified as such (in particular when faced with asymmetrical hyperfixations) (14,16,18). The development of coupled PET/scanner instruments should make it possible to reduce this risk of false positives by using PET-FDG/scanner fusion images (16), as described in other pathologies (20–22), by precisely locating these uptake sites on structures known to be responsible for variable physiological uptakes (20–22) (Fig. 1).

The variability of the results obtained in these studies can be partly explained by a variability in the criteria of recruitment. Indeed, in certain studies, the patients are regarded as presenting with a CUP only if the conventional assessment/work-up—including upper endoscopy with biopsies—is negative (12–14). In contrast, in other studies where upper

Table 1 Results Reported in the Main Studies Targeted on Cervical Lymph-Node Metastases

Authors	Year	Number of cases	Type	PD (%)	se	spe	vpp	vpn	ex	TI (%)
Rege et al. (5)	1994	4	NS	2 (50)	50	100	100	100	100	NE
Mukerji et al. (6)	1996	18	NS	9 (50)	81	38	64	60	np	NE
Braams et al. (7)	1997	13	NS	4 (30)	80	100	100	88	92	NE
Hanasono et al. (8)	1999	20	R	7 (35)	70	60	63	66	65	NE
Aassar et al. (9)	1999	17	NS	9 (52)	100	62	75	100	82	NE
Stokkel et al. (10)	1999	10	NS	6 (60)	100	25	66	100	60	6 (60)
Greven et al. (11)	1999	13	P	1 (7)	50	45	14	83	46	NE
Safa et al. (12)	1999	14	NS	3 (21)	75	90	100	90	92	NE
Jungehülsing et al. (13)	2000	27	NS	7 (25)	78	100	100	90	93	8 (29)
Bohuslavizki et al. (14)	2000	43	R	15 (34)	100	78	71	100	86	NE
Regelink et al. (15)	2002	50	R	16 (32)	100	94	89	100	np	10 (20)
Johansen et al. (16)	2002	42	P	10 (24)	90	67	50	95	73	10 (24)
Wong and Saunders (17)	2003	17	R	8 (47)	62	66	62	62	—	17 (53)
Stoeckli et al. (18)	2003	18	P	5 (27)	63	90	83	75	78	NE

Abbreviations: P, prospective study; R, retrospective study; PD, number of primaries detected (with percentage in brackets); se, sensitivity; spe, specificity; vpp, positive predictive value; vpn, negative predictive value; ex, accuracy; TI, number of patients for which PET-FDG had a therapeutic impact (with percentage given in brackets); NS, not specified; NE, not evaluated.

endoscopy does not form part of the conventional assessment, the patients are regarded as having a CUP before the upper endoscopy is carried out (10,11,15). This distinction is clearly important in evaluating the performances of PET-FDG. Indeed, in the study of Regelink et al. (15), PET-FDG allowed an identification of the primary in 16 out of 50 patients (identification percentage = 16/50, i.e., 35%), while upper endoscopy led to the identification of 12 cases. If we consider those patients with a negative upper endoscopy as having a CUP, this corresponds to an identification of primaries in 4 cases out of 38 (i.e., 10%) when based on PET-FDG. However, it clearly emerges from several studies that PET-FDG should be proposed at an early stage, i.e., before performing the upper endoscopy, thus directing the biopsies onto the suspect zones of uptake (6,10,15,18). In the study of Mukherji et al. (6), PET-FDG led to a doubling of the diagnostic output of the upper endoscopies.

In addition to identifying primaries, PET-FDG makes it possible to discover metastases that have so far not been diagnosed for a certain number of patients (10,13). Indeed, PET-FDG revealed the presence of additional metastases in 5 patients out of 10 according to Stokkel et al. (10), 7 patients out of 27 according to Jungehülsing et al. (13), and 6 patients out of 50 according to Regelink et al. (15).

The impact of PET-FDG on the therapeutic care of patients presenting with cervical metastases of unknown primary, which represents the most relevant information for evaluating the benefit of an examination, has only been reported in 5 studies out of 14 studies mentioned earlier (10,13,15,16,18) and in a sixth study reported by Rades et al. (19) that did not focus mainly on cervical metastases. PET-FDG thus led to a therapeutic modification of 20% to 60% of the examined patients. By pooling the results of the six studies, we can see that PET-FDG has a therapeutic impact for 36% of the patients (61 patients out of 168), generally by allowing an identification of the primary tumor (10,13,16,18,19), but sometimes also by identifying metastases that were up to then undiagnosed (13,15,19). In fact, PET-FDG led to a change of treatment because of the detection of additional metastases in two cases out of eight according to Jungehülsing et al. (13) and in six cases out of ten according to of Regelink et al. (15). The changes in therapeutic approach produced by PET-FDG generally involve a modification of the areas of radiotherapy [$n = 7/9$ for Wong et al. (18), 7/10 for Johansen et al. (16), 3/8 for Jungehülsing et al. (13), 3/6 for Stokkel et al. (10)], but in some cases give an indication of surgical resection [alone or associated with radiotherapy, $n = 2/9$ for Wong et al. (17), 1/10 for Johansen et al. (16), 4/8 for Jungehülsing et al. (13), 4/6 for Stokkel et al. (10), 7/22 for Rades et al. (19)], or, more rarely, an indication of chemotherapy (10,19) or therapeutic abstention because of the detection of a massive extension (16).

(A)

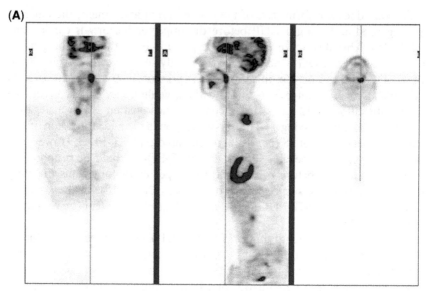

Frontal, sagittal, and transverse sections centered on the left tonsillar uptake

(B)

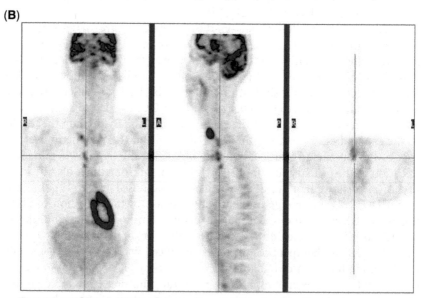

Frontal, sagittal, and transverse sections centered on the right laterotracheal uptakes

Figure 1   (*Caption on facing page.*)

PET-FDG AND CUP NOT TARGETED ON CERVICAL METASTASES

Table 2 summarizes the diagnostic performances of PET-FDG in the identification of a primary in patients having a CUP with various presentations (not targeted on cervical metastases). Eight studies have so far been published. One study, by Gupta et al., was targeted on cerebral metastases (25). Some of these studies included a variable proportion of patients with cervical metastases [13 patients out of 29 in the study of Kole et al. (23), which in addition included 8 melanomas, 11 patients out of 12 in the study of Lassen et al. (24), 2 patients out of 24 in the study of Lonneux and Reffad (26), 21 out of 42 in the study of Rades et al. (27), and 10 patients out of 25 in the study of Mantaka et al. (29)]. Moreover, the numbers of cases are low since the largest series only comprises 22 patients having CUP with a presentation other than cervical metastases (26). The patients were included if the primary was not identified clinically or after a negative result from a more or less full biological and radiological assessment. This contrasts with the study of Alberini et al., where the patients voluntarily underwent PET-FDG at a very early stage (if the clinical and biological examinations failed to locate a primary) with the aim of avoiding a costly diagnostic assessment (28). In this latter study, PET-FDG allowed the identification of a primary in 63% of patients and gave a higher performance than the conventional assessment in 27% of cases.

In these studies, PET-FDG allowed identification of the primary in 24% to 100% of the patients. If we analyze the results only for the patients with metastases other than cervical, excluding the study of Alberini et al. (28), where the PET-FDG was carried out at an early stage, and where the database for the patients does not allow such a distinction, it is found that PET-FDG led to an identification of the primary in 40 patients out of 75 (i.e., 53% of cases).

Figure 1 (*Figure on facing page*) Thirty-nine-year-old patient presenting with a CUP discovered when confronted with metastases located in the cerebral and left cervical lymphnode areas, having a histology in favor of an epidermoid carcinoma. The conventional assessment (i.e., full clinical examination including head and neck examination, cervical ultrasonography, and thoracic radiography) did not provide any orientation toward a primary. The PET-FDG reveals an intense left tonsillar hyperfixation evoking the primary site, as well as multiple hyperfixing lesions indicating metastases in the right and left cervical lymph nodes, and also in the right and left apical pleuro-pulmonary lymph nodes. The endoscopy performed during the decrease (**A**) confirmed the tonsillar lesion with a histology in favor of a poorly differentiated carcinoma, while the thoracic scan (**B**) performed in addition confirmed the existence of two apical sub-pleural lesions (*right* and *left*). The therapeutic care was made up of cerebral radiotherapy followed by chemotherapy. *Abbreviations*: CUP, carcinoma of an unknown primary site; PET-FDG, positron emission tomography with 18F-fluorodesoxyglucose.

Table 2 Results Reported in the Main Studies not Targeted on Cervical Lymph-Node Metastases

Authors	Year	Number of cases[a]	Type	PD (%)[a]	se	spe	vpp	vpn	ex	TI (%)[a]
Kole et al. (23)	1998	29	NS	7 (24)	70	100	100	86	89	3 (10)
		8		*3 (37)*						*1 (12)*
Lassen et al. (24)	1999	20	P	9 (45)	82	56	69	71	70	4 (20)
		9		*4 (44)*						*1 (11)*
Gupta et al. (25)	1999	12[b]	NS	12 (100)	100	100	100	NE	100	NE
Lonneux et al. (26)	2000	24	R	9 (37)	100	45	68	100	75	10 (42)
		22		*8 (36)*						
Bohuslavzki et al. (14)	2000	9	R	5 (55)	55	NE	100	NE	55	NE
Rades et al. (27)	2001	42	NS	26 (62)	100	NE	NE	100	NE	29 (69)
Alberini et al. (28)	2003	41	NS	26 (63)	92	100	100	80	94	11 (27)
Mantaka et al. (29)	2003	25	NS	12 (48)	100	61	70	100	80	11 (44)
		15		*8 (53)*						*8 (53)*

[a]Value for total population, and in italics for CUP other than cervical metastases.
[b]Targeted study in the case of suspected cerebral metastases of unknown primary.
Abbreviations: P, prospective study; R, retrospective study; PD, number of primaries detected (with percentage in brackets); se, sensitivity; spe, specificity; vpp, positive predictive value; vpn, negative predictive value; ex, accuracy; TI, number of patients for which PET-FDG had a therapeutic impact (with percentage given in brackets); NS, not specified; NE, not evaluated.

Once it is found, the primary is often localized in the lungs [$n = 4/4$ for Lassen et al. (24), 3/5 for Bohuslavizki et al. (14), 16/26 for Alberini et al. (28), 3/8 for Mantaka et al. (29), and 0/3 for Kole et al. (23)]. These results are probably overestimated since thoracic scans were not performed for all the patients. Furthermore, even when such scans were carried out, the acquisition and interpretation parameters were not specified. Indeed, in the study of Alberini et al., where scanner and pulmonary radiography were systematic, 16 pulmonary cancers were identified by PET-FDG, 12 by scanner, and only 3 by pulmonary radiography (28). Moreover, the author reports clearly that the conditions of interpretation of the thoracic scanners, produced by various radiologists in different centres, were worse than that for PET-FDG, which were reinterpreted by a group of experienced nuclear medicine specialists.

Otherwise, PET-FDG revealed the presence of additional metastases for 5 patients out of 29 in the study of Kole et al. (23), 4 patients out of 20 in the study of Lassen et al. (24), 7 patients out of 24 in the study of Lonneux et al. (26), 7 patients out of 9 in the study of Bohuslavizki et al. (14) and 13 patients out of 15 in the study of Mantaka et al. (29). In the study of Rades et al. dissemination of CUP was detected by FDG-PET alone, despite negative results of various preceding diagnostic procedures (27).

The therapeutic impact was evaluated in six studies (1,9,23,24,26,27,29) PET-FDG examinations conditioned the treatment for 11% to 69% of the patients, according to the series in question (19,23,24,26,27,29). These results are rather disparate, since two of the studies indicate a weak therapeutic impact, [11% and 12% (23,24)], and three others show a major therapeutic impact [42%, 53%, and 69% (26,27,29)]. By collating the results of these five studies, we find that PET-FDG modified the care of 57 patients out of 105 (i.e., 54%). The most commonly encountered modifications involve a change of the initially considered chemotherapy.

CONCLUSIONS

There are very few current data on the role of PET-FDG in the care of patients presenting with a CUP.

If the primary tumor is identified by FDG-PET without simultaneous dissemination, curative treatment can be administered. For patients with localized disease, the one-year survival is better, if the primary tumor has been detected by PET (100% vs. 73% if the primary tumor was not detected) (19,26). If dissemination is detected by FDG-PET alone after being missed by conventional diagnostic procedures, curative treatment concepts have to be replaced by palliative approaches. If dissemination is present at first diagnosis, the PET result has no impact on the treatment concept (19,26).

The most intensively explored situation is the form of cancer in patients presenting with cervical metastases of unknown primary. In such a situation,

PET-FDG makes it possible to locate a primary in 33% of the patients and leads to a therapeutic modification for 36% of the patients. This examination should be carried out before the upper endoscopy, thus guiding the biopsies if possible. PET-FDG has been very little explored for patients presenting with metastases that are not cervical. On the basis of the small amount of data available, PET-FDG in this indication appears to localize the primary in 53% of cases, with an impact on the therapeutic care for 35% of the patients.

These results should be taken into account with prudence, in particular for forms other than cervical metastases, because of the small number of published studies, which are often of retrospective character, as well as the small number of patients included. Moreover, there is some inhomogeneity in the definition of CUP and the methods for interpreting the conventional assessment and PET-FDG examinations.

The role of PET-FDG in the care of cancers of unknown primary site is defined by the SOR as follows: although it is not possible to define a standard, PET-FDG can be indicated in the search for a primary tumor in cases of cervical metastatic adenopathy without a known primary cancer, while supplementary and methodologically adapted studies are necessary to specify the role of this examination in such an indication (30).

REFERENCES

1. Warburg O. The Metabolism of Tumors. New York: Smith RR, 1931:129–169.
2. Hatanaka M. Transport of sugar in tumor cell membranes. Biochem Biophys Acta 1974; 355:77–104.
3. Rigo P, Paulus P, Kaschten BJ, et al. Oncological applications of positron emission tomography with fluorine-18 fluorodeoxyglucose. Eur J Nucl Med 1996; 23:1641–1674.
4. Maublant J, Vuillez JP, Talbot JN, et al. Tomographie par emission de positons (TEP) et F-18-fluorodesoxyglucose (FDG) en cancerology. Bull Cancer 1998; 85:935–950.
5. Rege S, Maass A, Chaiken L, et al. Use of positron emission tomography with fluorodeoxyglucose in patients with extracranial head and neck cancer. Cancer 1994; 73:3047–3058.
6. Mukherji SK, Drane WE, Mancuso AA, Parsons JT, Mendenhall WM, Stringer S. Occult primary tumors of the head and neck: detection with 2-(F-18) fluoro-2-deoxy-D-glucose SPECT. Radiology 1996; 199:761–766.
7. Braams JW, Pruim J, Kole AC, et al. Detection of unknown primary head and neck tumors by positron emission tomography. Int J Oral Maxillofac Surg 1997; 26:112–115.
8. Hanasono MM, Kunda LD, Segall GM, Ku GH, Terris DJ. Uses and limitations of FDG positron emission tomography in patients with head and neck cancer. Laryngoscope 1999; 109:880–885.
9. Aassar OS, Fischbein NJ, Caputo GR, et al. Metastatic head and neck cancer: role and usefulness of FDG PET in locating occult primary tumors. Radiology 1999; 210:177–181.

10. Stokkel MPM, Terhaard CH, Hordijk GJ, van Rijk PP. The detection of unknown primary tumors in patients with cervical metastases by dual-head positron emission tomography. Oral Oncology 1999; 35:390–394.
11. Greven KM, Keyes JW, William TJ, McGuirt WF, Joyce WT. Occult primary tumors of the head and neck. Lack of benefit from positron emission tomography imaging with 2-(F-18)fluoro-2-deoxy-D-glucose. Cancer 1999; 86:114–118.
12. Safa AA, Tran LM, Rege S, et al. The role of positron emission tomography in occult primary head and neck cancers. Cancer J Sci Am 1999; 5:214–218.
13. Jungehülsing M, Scheidhauer K, Damm M, et al. 2-(F18)-fluoro-2-deoxy-D-glucose positron emission tomography is a sensitive tool for the detection of occult primary cancer (carcinoma of unknown primary syndrome) with head and neck lymph node manifestation. Otolaryngol Head Neck Surg 2000; 123:294–301.
14. Bohuslavizki KH, Klutmann S, Kröger S, et al. FDG PET detection of unknown primary tumors. J Nucl Med 2000; 41:816–822.
15. Regelink G, Brouwer J, de Bree R, et al. Detection of unknown primary tumors and distant metastases in patients with cervical metastases: value of FDG-PET versus conventional modalities. Eur J Nucl Med 2002; 29:1024–1030.
16. Johansen J, Eigtved A, Buchwald C, Theilgaard SA, Hansen HS. Implication of F18-fluoro-2-deoxy-D-glucose positron emission tomography on management of carcinoma of unknown primary in the head and neck: a Danish cohort study. Laryngoscope 2002; 112:2009–2014.
17. Wong WL, Saunders M. The impact of FDG PET on the management of primary of occult primary head and neck tumors. Clin Oncol (R Coll Radiol) 2003; 15(8):461–466.
18. Stoeckli SJ, Mosna-Firlejczk K, Goerres GW. Lymph node metastases of squamous cell carcinoma from an unknown primary: impact of positron emission tomography. Eur J Nucl Med 2003; 30:441–416.
19. Rades D, Kuhnel G, Wildfang I, Borner AR, Knapp W, Karstens JH. The value of positron emission tomography (PET) for therapeutic management in patients with cancer of unknown primary (CUP). Strahlenther Onkol 2001; 177:525–529.
20. Garin E, Devillers A, Prigent F, et al. Acquisitions simultanées TEP/scanner: apport chez les patients suspect de récidive de cancer colo-rectal. Médecine Nucléaire imagerie fonctionnelle et métabolique 2003; 12:665–675.
21. Kluetz PG, Meltzer CC, Villemagne VL, et al. Combined PET/CT imaging in oncology impact on patient management. Clin Positron Imaging 2000; 3: 223–230.
22. Heller MT, Meltzer CC, Fukui MB, et al. Superphysiologic FDG uptake in the non-paralyzed vocal cord: resolution of a false positive PET result with combined PET-CT imaging. Clin Positron Imag 2000; 3:207–211.
23. Kole AC, Nieweg OE, Pruim J, et al. Detection of unknown primary tumors using positron emission tomography. Cancer 1998; 82:1160–1166.
24. Lassen U, Daugaard G, Eigtved A, Damgaard K, Friberg L. 18F-FDG whole body positron emission tomography (PET) in patients with unknown primary tumors (UPT). Eur J Cancer 1999; 35(7):1076–1082.
25. Gupta NC, Nicholson P, Bloomfield SM. FDG-PET in the staging work-up of patients with suspected intracranial metastatic tumors. Ann Surg 1999; 230(2): 202–206.

26. Lonneux M, Reffad AM. Metastases from unknown primary tumor: PET-FDG as initial staging procedure. Clin Positron Imag 2000; 3(4):137–141.
27. Rades D, Külnel G, Wildfang I, Börner AR, Schmoll HJ, Knapp W. Localised disease in cancer of unknown primary (CUP): the value of positron emission tomography (PET) for individual therapeutic management. Ann Oncol 2001; 12:1605–1609.
28. Alberini JL, Belhocine T, Hustinx R, Daenen F, Rigo P. Whole-body positron emission tomography using fluorodeoxyglucose in patients with metastases of unknown primary tumors (CUP syndrome). Nucl Med Comm 2003; 24: 1081–1086.
29. Mantaka P, Baum RP, Hertel A, Adams S, Nissen A, Sengupta S, Hör G. PET with 2-(F-18)6fluoro-2-Deoxy-d-glucose (FDG) in patients with cancer of unknown primary (CUP): influence on patients'diagnostic and therapeutic management. Cancer Biother Radiopharm 2003; 18:47–58.
30. Bourguet P et le groupe de travail pour l'élaboration des SOR pour l'utilisation de la TEP-FDG en cancérologie. Résultats dans ces cancers de site primitif inconnu. Bull Cancer 2003; 90:S103.

PROGNOSTIC FACTORS

6

Prognostic Considerations in Patients with Unknown Primary Carcinoma

Renato Lenzi

Department of Gastrointestinal Medical Oncology, The University of Texas M.D. Anderson Cancer Center, Houston, Texas, U.S.A.

Stéphane Culine

Centre Val d'Aurelle, Montpellier, France

INTRODUCTION

For the vast majority of patients with unknown primary carcinoma (UPC), well defined clinico-pathologic characteristics allowing accurate prognostic are not immediately evident and the identification of reliable prognostic indicators has proven challenging. Only in small numbers of patients the overall similarity of the clinical presentations to that of known primary cancers at a similar stage has resulted in the identification of subsets of patients with clinical and pathological features requiring specific guidelines that may translate into prolonged survival.

The importance of accurate prognostic information in the care of cancer patients cannot be overemphasized. The availability of reliable prognostic indicators helps provide patients with an insight into the likely course of their condition, allowing them to better make informed decisions. For the oncologist, prognostic considerations affect the choice of treatment; not infrequently the recommendation of whether to proceed with chemotherapy or supportive care only is largely based on prognostic considerations. For known primary cancers, detailed prognostic information is available based on the primary of origin and on other parameters including stage, demographic data such as age and sex, involved organ sites, performance status (PS), histology, and biologic markers. Such information is usually refined over time through the identification of new clinical or biological correlates of response and survival defining progressively more homogeneous cohorts of patients. By allowing a greater homogeneity of the patient populations studied, selection or stratification of patients according to reliable prognostic parameters contributes to the reproducibility of the results of clinical trials.

In patients with UPC, the main parameter generally used to define a homogeneous population of oncology patients, the primary tumor of origin, is not known. The frequency distribution of the primary types presenting as UPC is also not known and may not parallel the frequency of the known primaries in the overall population of cancer patients (1). The organ sites involved by metastatic disease of unknown origin do not appear to always follow the patterns common in known primary cancers (1). Therefore, it is difficult for most of the presentations of UPC to identify commonalities with those of known primary cancers and to choose a treatment approach based on similarities in the presentations.

For the vast majority of patients with UPC, well-defined clinico-pathologic characteristics allowing reasonably accurate prognostic and therapeutic subgrouping are not immediately evident, and the identification of reliable prognostic indicators has proven challenging. In fact, only in small numbers of patients the overall similarity of the clinical UPC presentations to that of known primary cancers at a similar stage has resulted in the identification of subsets of UPC patients. These subsets include women with axillary node metastases (2–4), women with peritoneal carcinomatosis and serous-papillary histology (5,6), patients with squamous cell carcinoma in cervical nodes (7), young men with the "extragonadal germ cell cancer syndrome" (8–10) of poorly differentiated cancer (PDC) histology, midline (mediastinal/retroperitoneal) and lymph node disease sites, and in some patients by the elevation of the β subunit of human chorionic gonadotropin (β-HCG) and/or of α-fetoprotein (AFP) in plasma or positivity by immunohistochemistry. For the majority of patients who do not fall into one of these rather favorable subsets, a number of studies with multivariate analyses identified poor PS, liver metastases, and abnormal serum lactate dehydrogenase (LDH) levels as the main recurrent adverse prognosticators. No international consensus has been defined. The knowledge of prognostic factors may help the oncologist to refine the daily management of patients to assess the results and to design clinical research studies. The assumptions concerning the type of the occult primary in some of these patient subgroups are supported by a similar prognosis, clinical course, and high response rates to treatments appropriate for the putative primary of origin, histological and biological characteristics, and occasional observations of the metachronous appearance of the primary (2,4,11,12). Additional UPC subsets with higher rates of response to chemotherapy and longer survival have been described based on a combination of histologic characteristics and response to platinum-based chemotherapy. They include patients with poorly differentiated neuroendocrine carcinomas (13,14) and the evolving group of patients with PDC and poorly differentiated adenocarcinoma (PDA) histology. While the median survival for UPC is of approximately 7 to 11 months, with less than 2% of the patients alive at five years (15–17), survival in patients belonging to these subgroups has been reported to be frequently measured in years.

PROGNOSTIC FACTORS IN UPC PATIENTS WITH PDC AND PDA

The initial description of a favorable prognosis subgroup of PDC and PDA patients initially included a small set of patients with common characteristics of male sex, young age, PDC or PDA histology, tumor involvement of lungs, mediastinum, retroperitoneum, and peripheral lymph nodes, elevated levels of AFP and/or β-HCG, and positive immunohistochemistry for these markers. The clinical course of these patients was characterized by a high rate of response to chemotherapy and by prolonged recurrence-free survival. The underlying primary was deemed to be a germ cell tumor, and this presentation was named the "unrecognized extragonadal germ cell tumor syndrome." Subsequently, a series was described of 71 unknown primary patients with PDC histology of which 62 were treated with a cisplatin-based regimen. A complete response rate of 22% was observed. Tumor location in peripheral lymph nodes, mediastinum, and retroperitoneum was significantly associated with favorable treatment outcome, with the underlying primary deemed to be a germ cell tumor. Treatment with a platinum-based regimen was advocated for all UPC patients with PDC histology, especially if peripheral lymph nodes, retroperitoneum, or mediastinum were involved (9).

With the increasing use of immunohistochemistry techniques for the evaluation of clinical biopsy material, however, it became apparent that several of the patients diagnosed with PDCs of unknown primary on morphological grounds only (and who had complete responses to platinum-based chemotherapy) had instead other malignancies such as lymphoma, melanoma, and germ cell tumors (18).

Hainsworth et al. (19) studied a prospectively compiled series of 220 patients treated with cisplatin-based chemotherapy over a period of 12 years. The median age was 39 years; 166 patients were males and 54 females. ECOG PS was zero to one in 188 patients and two to three in 32. In 48% of the patients, mediastinum, retroperitoneum, or peripheral lymph nodes were the dominant site of disease. Histologies after initial assessment by morphology on light microscopy were PDC (142 patients), PDA (51 patients), PDC with neuroendocrine features (12), and poorly differentiated malignant neoplasm (4 patients). In certain patients, pathological diagnoses were revised at different intervals after study entry based on additional information obtained after rebiopsy, at autopsy, and after retrospective pathology evaluation including immunohistochemistry. The definitive diagnoses were PDC, 97 patients; PDA, 70 patients; PDC with neuroendocrine features, 25 patients; melanoma, 8 patients; lymphoma 6 patients; poorly differentiated squamous cell carcinoma and sarcoma, 5 patients each; and yolk sac tumor, peripheral neuroepithelioma, mixed PDA/neuroendocrine carcinoma, and adenocarcinoma of the prostate, 1 each. Chemotherapy regimens varied during the period of accrual but all were cisplatin-based. Other drugs used were etoposide, bleomycin, vinblastin, ifosfamide, and doxorubicin. The majority of patients (209) received at least two courses of chemotherapy and were evaluated for response. The remainder were considered nonresponders. All patients were included in the survival calculations. The overall response rate was 62% with 26% complete responders. Median survival was 12 months with a 12-year survival of 16%.

The authors analyzed the correlation of eight clinical and pathologic variables with favorable responses to chemotherapy (complete response and disease-free survival) (Table 1). At age greater than 35 years, more than two sites of metastases, metastatic sites other than retroperitoneal or peripheral lymph nodes, elevated LDH, history of smoking more than 10 pack-years had a significant correlation with unfavorable response to chemotherapy. Elevated carcinoembryonic antigen (CEA) was significantly correlated with unfavorable outcome by univariate but not by multivariate analysis.

van der Gaast et al. studied 77 eligible previously untreated patients enrolled in two consecutive chemotherapy trials of BEP (cisplatin, bleomycin, intravenous etoposide: 59 patients) and DDV/VP (cisplatin and oral etoposide: 18 patients) (20). The patients were required to have PDA or undifferentiated carcinoma histology. Histologies other than carcinoma or adenocarcinoma (such as lymphoma) and overt germ cell tumors were carefully excluded using morphology, immunohistochemistry, and electron microscopy. Patients with elevated serum levels of AFP and/or β-HCG were also excluded. Most patients met previously described diagnostic criteria of the advanced PDCs of unknown primary site syndrome described by Greco et al. (9). Median survival was eight months, the estimated survival rate at five years was 15%, and overall response rate was 42%. Five of the nine complete responders had metastases limited to the lymph nodes.

The authors evaluated demographic, clinical, and laboratory variables for their significance as prognostic factors. Univariate analysis identified PS, histology, bone metastases, liver metastases, level of alkaline phosphatase, and AST as significant predictors of survival, of which lower PS and higher than normal alkaline phosphatase retained significance as independent adverse variables on multivariate analysis (Table 1). On the basis of these findings, the authors were able to subdivide the study patients into three prognostic groups: a favorable prognostic group with PS of 0 and normal alkaline phosphatase (median survival >4 years, response rate 69%), an intermediate prognostic group with either PS > 0 or elevated alkaline phosphatase (median survival = 10 months, response rate 46%), and a poor prognostic group with PS > 0 and elevated alkaline phosphatase (median survival = 4 months, response rate 26%) (20).

To evaluate the prevalence of PDC and PDA in an unselected population of UPC patients and to estimate whether the favorable treatment response profile and survival of PDC/PDA patients could be confirmed in a large series of consecutive patients with UPC, Lenzi et al. (21) studied 957 unselected, consecutive UPC patients for whom a full pathologic evaluation was available. Noncarcinoma histology was carefully excluded. Lenzi found that 140 patients were diagnosed with PDC and 197 patients with PDA. The median ages were 60 years for PDC and 59 years for PDA. No significant difference was detected in the male/female ratio between the two groups. Median survival for PDC patients was 13 months and for PDA patients nine months, with PDC histology being statistically significant by univariate Cox analysis (Table 1). By multivariate analysis, however, there was no significant survival advantage to PDC histology. Patients with PDC and PDA were shown, by multivariate regression analysis, to have a prognosis similar to that of patients with non-PDC and adenocarcinoma, respectively. When data were analyzed by recursive partitioning classification and regression tree (CART) analysis, no split occurred on poor tumor differentiation, indicating that this characteristic was not an independent predictor of survival. AFP and β-HCG levels less than 3.4 mIU/mL and 2.8 ng/mL, respectively, predicted best survival duration for those patients in whom they were measured. Treatment with platinum-based regimens, non-platinum based regimens, and no chemotherapy had no demonstrable effect on survival. Important favorable determinants of survival in the PDC/PDA group were presence of lymph node involvement, female sex, less than three metastatic sites, carcinoma histology, and age ≤64 years.

Patients with neuroendocrine and squamous cell carcinomas of unknown primary had significantly longer survivals than patients with either PDC or PDA (26 and 22 months, respectively).

The findings of this study appear to be supported by the results of more recent phase II trials in which patients with both well-differentiated and poorly differentiated carcinoma histology were treated using the same platinum-based regimens. A study of carboplatin, paclitaxel, and etoposide conducted by Greco and Hainsworth included 30 patients with well-differentiated adenocarcinoma and 21 with PDA or PDC. Response rates were not significantly different (45% and 48%) in the two groups (22). In a study of carboplatin and paclitaxel in UPC, Briasoulis et al. included 45 patients with adenocarcinoma and 27 with undifferentiated carcinoma. Response rates were 40% and 37%, respectively (23).

Table 1 Prognostic Factors in PDC and PDA of Unknown Primary Site

Author (References)	Study type	No. of patients	Variable	Survival effect	
				Univariate analysis	Multivariate analysis
Hainsworth et al. (19)	Prospectively compiled patients treated with cisplatin-based chemotherapy	220	Age (≤35, >35)		Unfavorable[a]
			Sites of metastasis:		
			No. of sites (1–2, >2)	Unfavorable	Unfavorable
			Sites other than retroperitoneal or peripheral lymph nodes	Unfavorable	Unfavorable
			CEA:	Unfavorable[b]	
			LDH	Unfavorable[b]	Unfavorable
			History of smoking (≤10, >10 pack-years)	Unfavorable	Unfavorable
van der Gaast et al. (20)	Retrospective data, two consecutive clinical trials	77	Age (<50, ≥50)	None	
			Sex	None	
			PS (WHO) <1	Favorable	Favorable
			Chemotherapy (BEP[c], DDP/VP[d])	None	
			Histology:		
			Adenocarcinoma	Unfavorable	
			Carcinoma, undifferentiated	Favorable	

Reference	No. of patients	Variable		
Lenzi et al. (21)	337	Sites of metastasis		
		No. of sites (1, 2, >2):	None	Favorable
		Bone	Unfavorable	
		Liver	Unfavorable	
		Liver or bone	Unfavorable	
		Lung	None	
		Lymph nodes	None	
		Dominant metastasis site:		
		Lymph nodes, other	None	
		LDH[e]	None	Favorable[f]
Prospective data, consecutive patients with PDA and PDC in a population of 957 UPC patients		Alkaline phosphatase[e]	Favorable	Favorable[f]
		AST[e]	Favorable	None[f]
		Age (≤64)		None[f]
		Sex (female)		None[f]
		Chemotherapy:		
		Platinum-based		
		Non-platinum-based		
		No chemotherapy		
		Histology:		
		PDC, PDA	PDC favorable	None
		PDC, Carcinoma	None	None
		PDA, Adenocarcinoma	None	None

[a]Survival decreased with age >35 years.
[b]Survival decreased with more than normal level.
[c]Bleomycin, etoposide, cisplatin
[d]Cisplatin, oral etoposide
[e]<1.25 times normal
[f]CART analysis

Abbreviations: PDC, poorly differentiated cancer; PDA, poorly differentiated adenocarcinoma; LDH, lactate dehydrogenase; CEA, carcinoembryonic antigen; PS, performance status; UPC, unknown primary carcinoma.

PROGNOSTIC FACTORS IN THE GENERAL POPULATION OF UPC PATIENTS

Several clinical characteristics and laboratory parameters have been proposed as relevant prognostic variables in populations of UPC patients not selected for histology of PDA or PDC.

Kambhu et al. (17) enrolled 62 patients in a phase II study of mitomycin–c, vindesine, and adriamycin. Patients with anaplastic tumors and PDC of unclear lineage were excluded. Fifty-seven patients were evaluable for response and survival. Median survival was seven months; overall response rate was 30%, and 5% of the patients had a complete response. Prognostic variables studied were sex, age, PS, number of sites of metastatic disease, abdominal visceral metastases, or liver metastases (Table 2). Female sex was the only variable significantly associated with response. When controlling for gender, none of the other variables were significantly associated with response. Absence of visceral metastases below the diaphragm, absence of liver metastases and PS > 70% (Karnofsky) were associated with longer survival by chi-square tests but only presence of visceral metastases below the diaphragm was significantly related to (shorter) survival by Cox regression analysis.

Abbruzzese et al. (16) studied natural history and prognostic factors of 657 unselected, consecutive patients with UPC. Median survival was 11 months, with 1.5% of the patients surviving beyond five years. Univariate survival analysis identified four favorable characteristics: lymph node involvement, carcinoma, squamous carcinoma, and neuroendocrine carcinoma histology, and eight unfavorable characteristics: male sex, adenocarcinoma histology, brain, bone, liver, lung, pleural metastases, and number of metastatic sites (survival decreased with increasing number of metastatic sites) (Table 2). Age, race, skin, and peritoneal metastases did not significantly affect survival. Multivariate analysis identified lymph nodal, peritoneal metastases, and neuroendocrine histology as independent predictors of longer survival. Male sex, ascending number of metastatic sites, adenocarcinoma histology, and liver metastases were identified as unfavorable prognostic indicators. Supraclavicular node involvement was also identified as a significant negative prognostic factor. In an attempt to ascertain the possible influence of treatment on the survival of these patients, the effect of chemotherapy on the survival of patients with PDC or undifferentiated carcinoma (two patient subgroups that had been described as responsive to cisplatin-based chemotherapy) was retrospectively examined. Of these patients, 64 had received chemotherapy, including cisplatin-based chemotherapy, and 45 had not received chemotherapy as part of their treatment. No effect of chemotherapy on survival was detected in this group, and the authors concluded that chemotherapy was unlikely to have altered the natural history of the disease in the remainder of the patients.

Table 2 Prognostic Factors in the General Population with CUP

Author (References)	Study type	No. of patients	Variable	Survival effect	
				Univariate analysis	Multivariate analysis
Kambhu et al. (17)	Phase II trial	62	Sites of metastasis:		
			No. of sites (1–2, 3+)	None	
			Visceral metastasis below diaphragm	Unfavorable	Unfavorable
			Liver metastasis	Unfavorable	
Abbruzzese et al. (16)	Consecutive patients Prospective data collection	657	Age (20–70+, 5 groups)	None	
			Sex (male)	Unfavorable	Unfavorable
			Race (white, other)	None	
			Sites of metastasis:		
			No. of sites (1, 2, 3+)	Unfavorable[a]	Unfavorable[a]
			Brain	Unfavorable	
			Bone	Unfavorable	
			Liver	Unfavorable	Unfavorable
			Lymph nodes	Favorable	Favorable
			Axilla	Favorable	
			Supraclavicular	None	Unfavorable
			Lung	Unfavorable	
			Peritoneum	None	Favorable
			Pleura	Unfavorable	
			Skin	None	
			Histology:		
			Adenocarcinoma	Unfavorable	Unfavorable

(Continued)

Table 2 Prognostic Factors in the General Population with CUP (*Continued*)

Author (References)	Study type	No. of patients	Variable	Survival effect	
				Univariate analysis	Multivariate analysis
Culine et al. (25)	Consecutive patients, retrospective review. Prognostic model data were validated using an independent data set	150[b]	Carcinoma	Favorable	
			Squamous	Favorable	
			Neuroendocrine	Favorable	Favorable
			Clinical variables:		
			Age (<57, ≥57)	None	
			Sex (male/female)	None	
			PS (0–1, 2–3)	Unfavorable[c]	Unfavorable[c]
			Histology:		
			Adenocarcinoma	None	
			Adenocarcinoma, PD[d]	None	
			Carcinoma, PD[d]	None	
			Sites of metastasis:		
			No. of sites (1, 2, >2)	Unfavorable[e]	
			Bone	None	
			Brain	None	
			Lymph nodes		
			Cervical or	None	
			Supraclavicular		
			Retroperitoneal		
			Liver	Unfavorable	
			Lung	None	
			Mediastinum	None	

Pleura	None	
Peritoneum	None	
Biologic parameters[f]		
Alkaline phosphatase	Unfavorable[g]	
CEA	Unfavorable[g]	
CA 19-9	None	
CA 125	Unfavorable[g]	
CA 15-3	None	
LDH	Unfavorable[g]	Unfavorable
Combined clinical variables and biologic parameters		
PS (0–1, 2–3)	Unfavorable	
LDH	Unfavorable	
Liver metastasis	None	

[a]Survival decreased with more organ sites.
[b]Prognostic model data
[c]Survival decreased with PS > 1.
[d]PD, poorly differentiated
[e]Survival decreased with more than two sites of metastases.
[f]Expressed as ≤ normal level or > normal level
[g]Survival decreased with > normal level.
Abbreviations: CUP, carcinoma of unknown primary site; PS, performance status; LDH, lactate dehydrogenase; CEA, carcinoembryonic antigen.

Hess et al. (24) performed multivariate analysis on 1000 consecutive UPC patients using Cox proportional hazards regression analysis and recursive partitioning CART analysis. Twenty-six clinical variables including demographics (age, ethnicity, and sex), pathology characteristics (histology, and differentiation), number of metastatic organ sites, lymph nodal metastases, involvement of specific nodal and extranodal sites were evaluated. Median overall survival was 11 months and five-year survival was 11%. The CART program generated a default tree after determining the optimal first split (presence or absence of liver metastases). Terminal subgroups size was constrained to no less than 20 patients. Ten groups were generated. The group with the longest median survival (40 months) constituted 127 patients with one to two sites of metastases, histology other than adenocarcinoma, and no adrenal, bone, liver, or pleural metastases. The group with the second longest median survival (24 months) comprised 28 patients with liver metatases of neuroendocrine carcinoma. The shortest surviving groups, with median survival of five months, included 153 patients with age >61.5 years, histology other than neuroendocrine, liver involvement, and 23 patients with adrenal metastases. An additional, not previously described group, of 76 patients with pleural involvement and a median survival of nine months was also identified. Two alternative trees were then created using an initial split on histology and lymph node involvement, respectively. The groups generated by the split on histology were similar to those of the default tree. The groups generated by the split on lymph nodes included a best survival group of 99 patients with non-adenocarcinoma histology, one or two involved sites, and lymph node involvement (median survival of 45 months); the two groups with the shortest survival (five months) were characterized by non-neuroendocrine histology, liver involvement, no lymph node involvement (117 patients), and by adrenal involvement, lymph node involvement, and more than two sites of metastases (39 patients). This study confirmed, using a different methodology, the prognostic importance of previously described variables such as liver and lymph nodal metastases, tumor histology, and number of metastatic sites, and identified new patient subgroups with unfavorable prognosis.

Culine et al. (25) focused on the study of baseline characteristics of potential prognostic value for UPC patients not belonging to subgroups with defined treatment indications to develop and validate a prognostic model of practical utility in the design of clinical trials in UPC. The reference population comprised 150 consecutive patients retrospectively identified, of whom approximately one-third had been enrolled in clinical trials. Patients with a single resectable site of metastasis, women with adenocarcinoma and axillary node involvement, women with papillary serous peritoneal carcinoma, patients with squamous or neuroendocrine histology were not eligible. Independent prognostic factors were determined using Cox regression analysis removing nonsignificant variables using a stepwise selection procedure. Median patient age was 57 years, median survival was 7.5 months. Two-year survival rate was 11%. One hundred and forty patients received chemotherapy, and 86% of those received a platinum-based regimen. By univariate analysis, adverse prognostic factors were PS of 2 to 3, presence of liver metastases, and more than two metastatic sites. Poor PS and liver metastases were confirmed as independent significant prognostic variables by multivariate analysis. A prognostic model including a good risk group (no liver metastases and good PS), an intermediate risk group (one only of liver metastases or poor PS), and a poor risk group (poor PS and liver metastases) identified cohorts of patients with significantly different median survivals of 10.8, 6, and 2.4 months, respectively. The authors then evaluated biologic parameters obtained prior to treatment, of which elevated serum LDH levels was shown to retain independent significance after multivariate analysis. Multivariate analysis including clinical and biological parameters showed no independent prognostic value for liver metastases. PS 2 to 3 and elevated LDH levels retained significance. A second prognostic model including the two significant predictors was validated in an independent data set of 116 patients. Median survival for good and poor risk groups were significantly different at 12 and 7 months, with one-year survival rates of 53% and 23%. The longer survival observed for the poor prognosis group in the validation set compared with the reference population was attributed by the authors to lower representation in the validation set of patients with poor PS.

This strategy resulted in a simple and validated prognostic model with practical applicability in the design of clinical trials.

PROGNOSTIC FACTORS AND UPC CLINICAL TRIALS

Evaluation of the results of phase II trials and comparison of results of different trials can be difficult if a practical and reliable instrument to assess prognostic factors in the study population is not available. The prognostic profile of the patients population can affect trial results by introducing a source of variability that is unrelated to the treatment effect that the trial seeks to estimate. In a randomized trial of cisplatin in combination with gemcitabine or irinotecan in UPC, conducted by the French Study Group on carcinomas of unknown primary site, although response rates of 55% and of 38%, respectively were observed, median survivals were only eight and six months; 60% of the patients belonged to a poor prognosis group, possibly contributing to the short survival (26). In a study of carboplatin and taxol in UPC, with an overall response rate of 38.7%, the authors reported a response rate of only 15% for patients with liver, bone, or multiorgan involvement, while patients with peritoneal carcinomatosis had a response rate of 68.4% and patients with predominant nodal disease had a response rate of 47.8%. Overall median survival was 13%. In the group of patients with visceral or disseminated metastases survival was 10 and 15 months in the group of patients with lymph node disease (23). The majority of recent phase II trials conducted in UPC have attempted to reduce the heterogeneity of the study population by excluding patients belonging in well-defined clinico-pathologic subgroups with specific treatment indications and well-defined probability of response/survival differing from those expected in the general populations of UPC patients. These subgroups have included patients with clinical features resembling those of specific primaries of a defined anatomic site (breast, squamous carcinoma of the head and neck, and ovarian carcinoma) or with specific histology (neuroendocrine tumors) known to predict prolonged survival. Present understanding of the distribution of prognostic factors in UPC patients suggests that these subgroups quantitatively represent a small portion of the variability of UPC; their exclusion leaves unaddressed potential imbalances in important determinants of prognosis such as PS, sex, number of metastatic sites, and type of metastatic sites (lymph nodes, liver, and other visceral sites) and certain laboratory parameters LDH.

In other trials, patient enrollment has been restricted to specific patient subgroups (PDA and PDC) deemed to benefit from specific treatment (platinum-based chemotherapy) and to have a distinctly favorable prognosis in regard to treatment response and survival. With the routine use of immunohistochemistry as part of the clinical pathologic evaluation, patients that might in the past fit these criteria but who actually had undiagnosed malignancies with favorable prognosis (lymphoma and germ cell tumors) have become progressively less likely to be included under these categories. An apparent shift in the reported response and survival of PDC histologies towards that of their nonpoorly differentiated counterparts has occurred in more recent studies, bringing their prognosis under similar determinants to the overall population of UPC patients. As a result, in more recent trials these patients have generally been included in studies of chemotherapy regimens targeted to the broader population of UPC patients.

CONCLUSION

In UPC, the diagnostic uncertainty as to the nature of the primary cancer also affects the formulation of a prognosis. For a small minority of patients, the presence of clusters of clinical characteristics that are easily apparent upon routine clinical evaluation mirrors the presentation of specific primary cancers except for the absence of a demonstrable site of origin. For those patients the prognosis also tends to be similar to that of patients with the corresponding primary of similar stage, and treatment choices are usually straightforward. For the majority of the patients, who present with combinations of clinical characteristics not easily matched to any specific primary of origin, formulating a prognosis depends on the less intuitive process of rigorous statistical evaluation. Many of the studies addressing the identification of prognostic factors in UPC have evaluated relatively small numbers of selected patients. Larger studies of unselected, consecutive patients have not confirmed the relevance of some of the variables thus proposed (21,24). Prospective data collection on large numbers of consecutive unselected patients with UPC appears to be an indispensable prerequisite for the reliable identification of such factors. Utilizing exclusively patients entered in clinical trial for the determination of prognostic factors affecting survival tends to result in the underestimation of the role of certain variables that are selected on the basis of eligibility criteria. Conversely, unrecognized strong determinants of survival may offset treatment effect causing difficulties in correctly evaluating and comparing trial outcomes.

The results of reported studies suggest that the use of CART analysis for the evaluation of UPC patients has the potential to result in the definition of additional relevant prognostic subgroups. The limitations of the method that include difficulty in interpreting P values (requiring validation on independent data) and the possible failure to detect small linear effects (24) are offset by the ability of CART to identify homogeneous prognostic patient subgroups using direct clinical characteristics that are logically combined, and to provide individual estimates of survival probability based directly on clinical variables (24).

Ongoing and planned clinical trials led by the French National group designed around the prognostic model developed and validated by Culine et al. (25) will target the study of more aggressive treatment regimens to good prognosis of UPC patients and studies of low toxicity chemotherapy versus best supportive care only to subgroups with poor prognosis. More extensive use and prospective evaluation of CART-generated prognostic models may also help in the definition of less heterogeneous UPC populations more suitable for focused clinical trials. Studies of the basic biology of UPC aiming to identify specific molecular targets promise to also provide additional useful prognostic indicators. Use of gene profiling to compare known primary tumors with UPC may lead to an increase in the rate of identification of the primary site, thereby reducing the number of patients for whom the lack of a specific diagnosis contributes to prognostic uncertainty.

REFERENCES

1. Nystrom JS, Weiner JM, Heffelfinger-Juttner J, Irwin LE, Bateman JR, Wolf RM. Metastatic and histologic presentations in unknown primary cancer. Semin Oncol 1977; 4(1):53–58.
2. Ellerbroek N, Holmes F, Singletary E, Evans H, Oswald M, McNeese M. Treatment of patients with isolated axillary nodal metastases from an occult primary carcinoma consistent with breast origin. Cancer 1990; 66(7):1461–1467.
3. Copeland EM, McBride CM. Axillary metastases from unknown primary sites. Ann Surg 1973; 178(1):25–27.

4. Rosen PP, Kimmel M. Occult breast carcinoma presenting with axillary lymph node metastases: a follow-up study of 48 patients. Hum Pathol 1990; 21(5): 518–523.

5. Strnad CM, Grosh WW, Baxter J, et al. Peritoneal carcinomatosis of unknown primary site in women. A distinctive subset of adenocarcinoma. Ann Intern Med 1989; 111(3):213–217.

6. Ransom DT, Patel SR, Keeney GL, Malkasian GD, Edmonson JH. Papillary serous carcinoma of the peritoneum. A review of 33 cases treated with platin-based chemotherapy. Cancer 1990; 66(6):1091–1094.

7. Wang RC, Goepfert H, Barber AE, Wolf P. Unknown primary squamous cell carcinoma metastatic to the neck. Arch Otolaryngol Head Neck Surg 1990; 116(12):1388–1393.

8. Richardson RL, Schoumacher RA, Fer MF, et al. The unrecognized extragonadal germ cell cancer syndrome. Ann Intern Med 1981; 94(2):181–186.

9. Greco FA, Vaughn WK, Hainsworth JD. Advanced poorly differentiated carcinoma of unknown primary site: recognition of a treatable syndrome. Ann Intern Med 1986; 104(4):547–553.

10. Fox RM, Woods RL, Tattersall MH, McGovern VJ. Undifferentiated carcinoma in young men: the atypical teratoma syndrome. Lancet 1979; 1(8130): 1316–1318.

11. Rosen PP. Axillary lymph node metastases in patients with occult noninvasive breast carcinoma. Cancer 1980; 46(5):1298–1306.

12. Davidson BJ, Spiro RH, Patel S, Patel K, Shah JP. Cervical metastases of occult origin: the impact of combined modality therapy. Am J Surg 1994; 168(5):395–399.

13. Hainsworth JD, Johnson DH, Greco FA. Poorly differentiated neuroendocrine carcinoma of unknown primary site. A newly recognized clinicopathologic entity. Ann Intern Med 1988; 109(5):364–371.

14. Moertel CG, Kvols LK, O'Connell MJ, Rubin J. Treatment of neuroendocrine carcinomas with combined etoposide and cisplatin. Evidence of major therapeutic activity in the anaplastic variants of these neoplasms. Cancer 1991; 68(2): 227–232.

15. Pasterz R, Savaraj N, Burgess M. Prognostic factors in metastatic carcinoma of unknown primary. J Clin Oncol 1986; 4(11):1652–1657.

16. Abbruzzese JL, Abbruzzese MC, Hess KR, Raber MN, Lenzi R, Frost P. Unknown primary carcinoma: natural history and prognostic factors in 657 consecutive patients. J Clin Oncol 1994; 12(6):1272–1280.

17. Kambhu SA, Kelsen DP, Fiore J, et al. Metastatic adenocarcinomas of unknown primary site. Prognostic variables and treatment results. Am J Clin Oncol 1990; 13(1):55–60.

18. Hainsworth JD, Wright EP, Johnson DH, Davis BW, Greco FA. Poorly differentiated carcinoma of unknown primary site: clinical usefulness of immunoperoxidase staining. J Clin Oncol 1991; 9(11):1931–1938.

19. Hainsworth JD, Johnson DH, Greco FA. Cisplatin-based combination chemotherapy in the treatment of poorly differentiated carcinoma and poorly differentiated adenocarcinoma of unknown primary site: results of a 12-year experience. J Clin Oncol 1992; 10(6):912–922.

20. van der Gaast A, Verweij J, Planting AS, Hop WC, Stoter G. Simple prognostic model to predict survival in patients with undifferentiated carcinoma of unknown primary site. J Clin Oncol 1995; 13(7):1720–1725.

21. Lenzi R, Hess KR, Abbruzzese MC, Raber MN, Ordonez NG, Abbruzzese JL. Poorly differentiated carcinoma and poorly differentiated adenocarcinoma of unknown origin: favorable subsets of patients with unknown-primary carcinoma? J Clin Oncol 1997; 15(5):2056–2066.

22. Greco FA, Hainsworth JD. One-hour paclitaxel, carboplatin, and extended-schedule etoposide in the treatment of carcinoma of unknown primary site. Semin Oncol 1997; 24(6 suppl 19):S101–S105.

23. Briasoulis E, Kalofonos H, Bafaloukos D, et al. Carboplatin plus paclitaxel in unknown primary carcinoma: a phase II Hellenic Cooperative Oncology Group Study. J Clin Oncol 2000; 18(17):3101–3107.

24. Hess KR, Abbruzzese MC, Lenzi R, Raber MN, Abbruzzese JL. Classification and regression tree analysis of 1000 consecutive patients with unknown primary carcinoma. Clin Cancer Res 1999; 5(11):3403–3410.

25. Culine S, Kramar A, Saghatchian M, et al. Development and validation of a prognostic model to predict the length of survival in patients with carcinomas of an unknown primary site. J Clin Oncol 2002; 20(24):4679–4683.

26. Culine S, Lortholary A, Voigt JJ, et al. Cisplatin in combination with either gemcitabine or irinotecan in carcinomas of unknown primary site: results of a randomized phase II study-trial for the French Study Group on Carcinomas of Unknown Primary (GEFCAPI 01). J Clin Oncol 2003; 21(18):3479–3482.

7

Treatment of Patients with Favorable Subsets of Unknown Primary Carcinoma

John D. Hainsworth
Sarah Cannon Research Institute, Nashville, Tennessee, U.S.A.

INTRODUCTION

One of the major advances in the management and treatment of patients with unknown primary carcinoma has been the recognition of several favorable subsets within this heterogeneous group. Although patients who fit into one of these subsets comprise only a minority of the entire group, they can be identified on the basis of specific clinical or pathological features. Early recognition of these patients is important, because specific treatments can improve outcome and extend survival.

The appropriate initial evaluation for accurate recognition of these treatable subsets has been described in Chapter 4. In this chapter, the recommended treatments for each subset will be discussed, as well as expected outcome of patients. Since two of the treatable subsets (women with isolated axillary adenopathy and patients with squamous cancer involving cervical lymph nodes) are discussed in separate chapters, they will be briefly mentioned here.

WOMEN WITH PERITONEAL CARCINOMATOSIS

In women, adenocarcinoma causing diffuse peritoneal involvement usually originates in the ovary, although carcinomas arising in the gastrointestinal tract or breast can occasionally produce this syndrome. In one large study, 55% of women who presented with malignant ascites had a primary site identified in the ovary, while 25% had nongynecologic primary sites identified.

In the remaining 20% of women, no primary site could be identified at the time of laparotomy (1). In most patients with peritoneal carcinomatosis of unknown primary site, histologic features resemble ovarian carcinoma, with features such as papillary configuration or psammoma bodies. However, some patients have poorly differentiated carcinoma, analogous to poorly differentiated epithelial ovarian carcinoma. Serum levels of CA 125 are usually elevated. This syndrome occurs more frequently in women with BRCA-1 mutations, and occasionally develops in women from families at high risk for ovarian cancer even after prophylactic oophorectomy (2,3). When histologic features suggest ovarian carcinoma, this syndrome has been termed "multifocal extraovarian serous carcinoma" or "peritoneal papillary serous carcinoma."

Several case reports in the 1980s suggested excellent responses of patients with this syndrome when treated with chemotherapy effective against ovarian cancer. Subsequently, several reported series have better characterized the responsiveness of these patients. As summarized in Table 1, several investigators have documented high initial response rates with long-term remissions in 15% to 20% of patients (4–9). Chemotherapy regimens containing cisplatin and cyclophosphamide have been used most frequently; however, recent reports have documented the activity of platinum/paclitaxel regimens (9). As in ovarian cancer, most long-term remissions have been observed in patients who had successful surgical cytoreduction prior to receiving chemotherapy. The general acceptance of the chemosensitivity of patients in this group is now signified by the routine inclusion of such patients in clinical trials for advanced ovarian carcinoma.

In summary, women with metastatic adenocarcinoma involving the peritoneal surface have tumors that are distinct in biology and are often responsive to chemotherapy. Optimal management of these patients should

Table 1 Peritoneal Carcinomatosis in Women: Treatment Results

Investigator (References)	No. of patients	Chemotherapy	Response rate	5-year survival
Strnad et al. (4)	18	Cisplatin-based	39%	28% (3 yr)
Dalrymple et al. (5)	31	Cisplatin-based	32%	0
Ransom et al. (6)	33	Cisplatin-based	NR	20%
Fromm et al. (7)	44	Cisplatin/ cyclophosphamide	64%	22%
Bloss et al. (8)	33	PAC	64%	15%
Piver et al. (9)	46	PAC, TP	66%	NR

Abbreviations: C, cyclophosphamide; A, doxorubicin; P, cisplatin; T, paclitaxel; NR, not reported.

follow guidelines for stage III ovarian cancer, including initial maximal surgical cytoreduction if possible, followed by postoperative chemotherapy. Since taxane/platinum combinations have proved superior in advanced ovarian cancer (10,11), these regimens should also be employed for the treatment of women with peritoneal carcinomatosis.

The syndrome of peritoneal carcinomatosis with papillary serous histology and elevated serum CA 125 may also occur rarely in males (12). A similar management approach in these patients seems reasonable, particularly if tumor involvement is isolated to the peritoneum.

WOMEN WITH AXILLARY LYMPH NODE METASTASES

Metastatic breast cancer should be suspected in all women who are found to have metastatic adenocarcinoma involving axillary lymph nodes. The initial pathologic evaluation should include measurement of hormone receptor and HER2 status; elevated levels provide strong evidence for the diagnosis of breast cancer (13). Magnetic resonance imaging (MRI) and positron emission tomography (PET) scanning have aided in the identification of occult breast primary tumors, even after normal physical examination and mammography (14,15).

In patients who have no demonstrable breast primary, clinical management should follow guidelines for stage II breast cancer. Patients with involvement isolated to unilateral axillary lymph nodes have prognoses with treatment similar to patients with stage II breast cancer. The treatment of this well-recognized subgroup is detailed in Chapter 11.

ADENOCARCINOMA PRESENTING AS A SINGLE METASTATIC LESION

In occasional patients, only a single metastatic lesion can be identified even after a complete staging evaluation. Single lesions have been described in a variety of sites, including lymph nodes, brain, adrenal gland, lung, liver, and bone. The possibility of an unusual primary site mimicking a metastatic lesion should always be considered, but this possibility can usually be excluded on the basis of clinical or pathologic features. Prior to planning treatment, a PET scan is probably helpful in this patient group, primarily for the purposes of excluding other occult metastatic sites (16).

In most patients who present with a single metastatic lesion, other metastatic sites become evident within a relatively short time. However, definitive local treatment sometimes produces long disease-free intervals, and occasionally patients have prolonged survival. For example, in one report of patients presenting with isolated single brain metastases (a site in which the lesions were unquestionably metastases rather than unrecognized primary lesions), 15% of patients remained without evidence of other tumor progression five years after definitive resection of the brain metastasis (17). Therefore, the resection of the solitary lesion should be undertaken, if clinically feasible. In some instances, local radiation therapy may also be appropriate to maximize the chance of local control (17,18).

Following successful local treatment, the concept of employing "adjuvant" systemic chemotherapy is attractive. In isolated case reports, such patients have had long-term survival. However, there has been no systematic study of this issue, and proof of its superiority versus local treatment alone is lacking.

YOUNG MEN WITH FEATURES OF EXTRAGONADAL GERM CELL TUMOR

The diagnosis of extragonadal germ cell tumor should be suspected in young men who develop poorly differentiated carcinoma with involvement of the mediastinum or retroperitoneum. Lung metastases are also common in this group of patients. In this clinical setting, elevated levels of either HCG or α-fetoprotein add further evidence to support the diagnosis of extragonadal germ cell tumor. Since there are no immunoperoxidase stains that are entirely specific for germ cell tumors, this diagnosis sometimes remains in doubt after standard pathologic evaluation. Detection of the i(12p) chromosomal abnormality specific for germ cell tumors has confirmed the diagnosis of extragonadal germ cell tumor in some of these patients (19).

Since extragonadal germ cell tumors are potentially curable with cisplatin-based combination chemotherapy, young men with these clinical features should be managed according to standard guidelines for extragonadal germ cell tumors. Initial treatment should include a combination of cisplatin, etoposide, and bleomycin (20), or a regimen with proven equivalent efficacy. In patients who have a good response after four courses, but have residual radiographic abnormalities, definitive surgical resection should be considered if feasible.

Numerous case reports in small patient series have documented the high level of sensitivity of this group of patients, when treated with chemotherapy regimens active against germ cell tumors (19,21–25). From these small series, it is difficult to estimate the complete response rate in this patient group; however, patients with multiple clinical features of extragonadal germ cell tumors are most likely to respond well.

SQUAMOUS CARCINOMA INVOLVING CERVICAL LYMPH NODES

The cervical lymph nodes are the most common metastatic site for squamous cell carcinoma of unknown primary origin. Patients are usually middle aged or elderly and many have a history of tobacco and alcohol use. In most patients, unilateral involvement of upper or mid-cervical lymph nodes is evident at presentation. Optimal evaluation includes a thorough endoscopic evaluation of the oropharynx, hypopharynx, nasopharynx, larynx, and upper esophagus, with biopsy of all suspicious areas. Computed tomography (CT) of the neck and PET scanning are also useful in identifying primary sites in the head and neck, as well as precisely defining the extent of lymph node involvement. With such an evaluation, a primary site in the head and neck area is identified in approximately 85% of patients (26).

When a thorough clinical evaluation fails to reveal a primary site, these patients should be treated according to established guidelines for the management of locally advanced squamous carcinomas of the head and neck. A detailed discussion of treatment of this patient subset is presented in Chapter 10. The potential for long-term, disease-free survival in this patient subset has long been recognized, and has been documented in multiple series of patients (27–33). In recent years, combined modality therapy with concurrent radiation therapy and chemotherapy has improved the outcome for patients with locally advanced head and neck cancer. Such approaches also appear highly effective in patients with squamous carcinoma involving cervical lymph nodes; recent reports have documented long-term survival in the 50% to 60% range (32,33).

SQUAMOUS CARCINOMA INVOLVING INGUINAL LYMPH NODES

Most patients with squamous cell carcinoma involving inguinal lymph nodes have a detectable primary site in the genital or anorectal area. Digital rectal examination and anoscopy should be routinely performed to exclude lesions in the anorectal area. All women should undergo careful pelvic examination with biopsy of any suspicious areas. Identification of a primary site in these patients is important, since potentially curative therapy is available for carcinomas of the anus, vulva, vagina, and cervix, even after spread to regional lymph nodes.

For the occasional patient in whom no primary site is identified, definitive local therapy with inguinal lymph node dissection or radiation therapy can result in long-term survival (34). In recent years, combined modality therapy with concurrent chemotherapy and radiotherapy has improved prognosis for several of the primary cancers arising in this region (e.g., anus, cervix, and bladder). Owing to the rarity of squamous carcinoma of unknown primary site presenting in inguinal lymph nodes, systematic study of combined modality therapy for this syndrome has not been published. However, combined modality treatment with concurrent radiotherapy and platinum-based chemotherapy seems reasonable in such patients.

NEUROENDOCRINE CARCINOMA WITH AN UNKNOWN PRIMARY SITE

A broad spectrum of neuroendocrine carcinoma is now recognized, in part due to improved pathologic methods for making the diagnosis. Most well-described neuroendocrine tumors have indolent biology and typical histologic features (e.g., carcinoid tumors, islet cell tumors, and paraganglioma). A second group of neuroendocrine tumors, typified by small cell lung cancer, can be readily identified by light microscopy, and share an aggressive biology. A third group of neuroendocrine tumors, previously under-diagnosed, has high grade biology and no distinctive neuroendocrine features by light microscopy. In this group, the initial diagnosis is often "poorly differentiated carcinoma" or "poorly differentiated adenocarcinoma"; neuroendocrine features are recognized only after immunoperoxidase staining and/or electron microscopy is performed. Neuroendocrine tumors in each of these three categories can present with an unknown primary site. Since management differs substantially based on the expected tumor biology, these three categories of neuroendocrine tumors are considered separately.

Low-Grade Neuroendocrine Carcinoma

Metastatic low grade neuroendocrine carcinomas are occasionally found at metastatic sites without an obvious primary site. In such patients, the metastases almost always involve the liver; some patients have concurrent bone involvement. Some of these patients have clinical syndromes produced by tumor secretion of bioactive substances. Pathologic examination usually reveals easily recognizable neuroendocrine tumors with carcinoid or islet cell features and low mitotic activity. Occasionally, primary sites in the gastrointestinal tract or pancreas are subsequently identified during the clinical course.

Not surprisingly, these low-grade neuroendocrine tumors have an indolent biologic behavior, similar to other typical carcinoid tumors. These neoplasms are usually refractory to standard cytotoxic chemotherapy. However, as in other carcinoid or islet cell tumors, local therapy (resection of isolated metastases, hepatic artery chemoembolization, radiofrequency ablation) may provide substantial palliation by reducing tumor volume. In addition, treatment with somatostatin analogs may result in long periods of disease stability. 5-Fluorouracil-based chemotherapy produces occasional responses.

Small Cell Carcinoma

Patients with small cell anaplastic carcinoma at a metastatic site usually have a bronchogenic primary. CT of the chest should always be performed. In patients with risk factors for small cell lung cancer, fiberoptic bronchoscopy should also be considered. A large number of extrapulmonary primary sites have also been described (e.g., salivary gland, esophagus, bladder, prostate, ovary, and cervix). When a primary site is identified, these tumors have been collectively described as "extrapulmonary small cell carcinomas," although any molecular similarity to small cell lung cancer is doubtful. Patients with localizing symptoms should have appropriate diagnostic studies performed in an attempt to identify a primary site.

Patients with small cell anaplastic carcinomas of unknown primary site usually demonstrate a rapidly progressive clinical course. Many patients have multiple metastatic sites at the time of diagnosis. Unlike the low-grade, carcinoid-type neuroendocrine tumors, these tumors are responsive to chemotherapy, and all patients should be considered for a trial of treatment at the time of diagnosis. Although "optimum" chemotherapy regimens are not defined, combination regimens effective in the treatment of small cell lung cancer are currently recommended. For patients with a single site of tumor involvement, local radiation therapy in conjunction with chemotherapy should also be considered.

Poorly Differentiated Neuroendocrine Carcinoma

In 10% to 15% of poorly differentiated carcinomas of unknown primary site, immunoperoxidase staining or electron microscopy identifies neuroendocrine features. In some of these patients, neuroendocrine features are also suggested by light microscopic examination, whereas in others the light microscopic diagnosis is "poorly differentiated carcinoma." Patients with poorly differentiated neuroendocrine carcinomas have rapidly growing tumors with frequent widespread metastasis and poor prognoses. These neoplasms are rarely associated with clinical signs and symptoms produced by tumor secretion of bioactive substances.

Recognition of this patient subset is important, since poorly differentiated neuroendocrine carcinomas are often highly sensitive to combination chemotherapy. In a retrospective evaluation of 43 such patients treated within a larger group of patients with unknown primary cancer, Hainsworth and Greco documented objective responses in 33 of 43 evaluable patients (77%) when treated with platinum/etoposide-based regimens (35). Thirteen of these patients had complete responses, and eight remained continuously disease-free more than two years after completion of therapy. Other case reports have also documented long-term survival of patients with aggressive neuroendocrine tumors of unknown primary site who received platinum-based chemotherapy (36,37).

More recently, we have treated patients with poorly differentiated neuroendocrine carcinoma in a prospective clinical trial, evaluating the combination of paclitaxel, carboplatin, and etoposide (38). Preliminary results of this prospective trial have confirmed the chemosensitivity of many of these neoplasms. To date, 13 of 28 patients (46%) have had major responses, with a two-year survival of 38%.

The origin of these poorly differentiated neuroendocrine tumors remains unclear, but it is likely that the group is heterogeneous. Some patients may have small cell lung cancer with an "occult" primary site. However, the absence of a smoking history makes the diagnosis of a pulmonary primary unlikely in most patients. It is probable that some of these tumors are undifferentiated variants of carcinoid tumors, albeit without a recognizable primary site. Metastatic anaplastic neuroendocrine carcinomas of gastrointestinal origin ("anaplastic carcinoids") have also demonstrated sensitivity to platinum-based chemotherapy (39).

Although the nature of these tumors remains undefined, patients with poorly differentiated neuroendocrine carcinoma often respond well to chemotherapy, and all patients in this group should be considered for an empiric trial of a platinum/etoposide-based regimen. In patients with a single tumor site, local treatment (either surgical resection or radiation therapy) should be considered in addition to combination chemotherapy.

POORLY DIFFERENTIATED CARCINOMA

The treatment and prognosis of patients with poorly differentiated carcinoma of unknown primary site who lack characteristics of extragonadal germ cell tumor remains controversial. Whether these patients represent a distinct, treatable subset is questionable. In a group of 220 patients prospectively identified and treated between 1978 and 1989, Hainsworth and Greco reported a 62% overall response rate with 26% complete responses (25). These patients received treatment with intensive cisplatin-based combination regimens used in the treatment of advanced testicular cancer. A minority of patients (14%) were tumor-free after a minimum follow-up of eight years (40). Although this was a select group of patients, as evidenced by median age of 39 years, few patients had clinical characteristics strongly suggestive of extragonadal germ cell tumor. Clinical features predictive of a favorable treatment outcome included tumor location in the retroperitoneum or peripheral lymph nodes, fewer sites of metastases, younger age, and a negative smoking history (25). However, elevation of serum tumor marker HCG and AFP in the absence of other clinical features of extragonadal germ cell tumor has not been predictive of chemotherapy responsiveness in subsequent experience (41).

In contrast to this experience, the group at M.D. Anderson could not identify a subset of patients with poorly differentiated carcinoma who experienced long-term survival following chemotherapy (42). In a large group of patients receiving a wide variety of treatments, no long-term survivors were identified, and poorly differentiated carcinoma patients had similar outcomes when compared with those with adenocarcinoma. However, several of the same clinical features were found to be predictive of clinical

Table 2 Summary of Treatable Subsets

Subset	Histology	Additional pathologic evaluation	Additional clinical evaluation	Treatment
Women, peritoneal carcinomatosis	Adenocarcinoma, PDC	—	CA 125	Treat as stage III ovarian carcinoma
Women, axillary adenopathy	Adenocarcinoma, PDC	ER/PR, HER-2	MRI breast PET scan	Treat as stage II breast cancer
Single metastasis	Adenocarcinoma, PDC	—	—	Definitive local treatment
Extragonadal germ cell tumor features	PDC	Consider molecular genetic analysis	HCG, AFP	Treat as extragonadal germ cell tumor
Cervical adenopathy	Squamous	—	ENT endoscopy, PET scan	Treat as locally advanced head/neck cancer
Inguinal adenopathy	Squamous	—	Sigmoidoscopy, PET scan	Definitive local therapy. Consider concurrent platinum-based chemotherapy
Neuroendocrine carcinoma, well differentiated	—	—	—	Treat as metastatic carcinoid tumor
Neuroendocrine carcinoma, small cell anaplastic or poorly differentiated	—	Chromogranin, synaptophysin stains	—	Treat with platinum/etoposide-based regimen

Abbreviations: MRI, magnetic resonance imaging; PDC, poorly differentiated carcinoma; PET, positron emission tomography.

response, including tumor location in lymph nodes, fewer metastatic sites, young age, and female sex.

Lastly, the group of Institut Gustave Roussy, Villejuif, France, performed a prospective study in which patients with a carcinoma of an unknown primary which did not fit into one of the favorable subsets described in this chapter were treated differently according to pathological differentiation: a cisplatin–etoposide association in poorly differentiated carcinomas and a cisplatin and 5-fluorouracil association in well- or moderately well-differentiated carcinomas (43). In this study, no obvious survival difference was seen between the two groups.

At present, a trial of combination chemotherapy should be considered for most patients with poorly differentiated carcinoma of unknown primary site. As previously discussed, patients with clinical features of extragonadal germ cell tumors should receive intensive cisplatin-based chemotherapy with a regimen used for the treatment of germ cell tumors. For other patients in this group who have good performance status, a trial of platinum-based chemotherapy should also be considered. We have recently included these patients in clinical trials evaluating empiric platinum/taxane regimens.

CONCLUSION

Table 2 provides a summary of the various treatable subsets of patients described in this chapter, with brief treatment recommendations. For several of these subsets, recommendations for treatment parallel the treatment of specific carcinomas of known primary site. As treatment evolves and improves for these cancers, the treatment approach for the much less common unknown primary counterparts should also change. Since many of these subsets are relatively rare, it is unlikely that definitive treatment series will be available to substantiate the advantages of such treatment changes. Ultimately, better treatment of unknown primary cancer will parallel improvements in treatment for more common advanced solid tumors, particularly those of lung and gastrointestinal origin. With the recent vastly improved understanding of the malignant process, and the introduction of a variety of targeted agents, further advances in the near future seem likely.

REFERENCES

1. Wilailak S, Linasmita V, Srivannaboon S. Malignant ascites in female patients: a seven-year review. J Med Assoc Thai 1999; 82:15.
2. Schorge JO, Muto MG, Welch WR, et al. Molecular evidence for multifocal papillary serous carcinoma of the peritoneum in patients with germ-line BRCA1 mutations. J Natl Cancer Inst 1998; 90:841.

3. Tobacman JK, Greene MH, Tucker MA, et al. Intra-abdominal carcinomatosis after prophylactic oophorectomy in ovarian cancer-prone families. Lancet 1982; 2:795.
4. Strnad CM, Grosh WW, Baxter J, et al. Peritoneal carcinomatosis of unknown primary site in women. Ann Intern Med 1989; 111:213–217.
5. Dalrymple JC, Bannatyne P, Russell P, et al. Extraovarian peritoneal serous papillary carcinoma. A clinicopathologic study of 31 cases. Cancer 1989; 64:110–115.
6. Ransom DT, Patel SR, Kenney GL, et al. Papillary serous carcinoma of the peritoneum: a review of 33 cases treated with cisplatin-based chemotherapy. Cancer 1990; 66:1091–1094.
7. Fromm GL, Gershenson DM, Silva EG. Papillary serous carcinoma of the peritoneum. Obstet Gynecol 1990; 75:75–79.
8. Bloss JD, Liao SY, Buller RE, et al. Extraovarian peritoneal serous papillary carcinoma: a case–control retrospective comparison to papillary adenocarcinoma of the ovary. Gynecol Oncol 1993; 50:347–351.
9. Piver MS, Eltabbakh GH, Hempling RE, et al. Two sequential studies for primary peritoneal carcinoma: induction with weekly cisplatin followed by either cisplatin/doxorubicin/cyclophosphamide or paclitaxel/cisplatin. Gynecol Oncol 1997; 67:141–146.
10. McGuire WP, Hoskins WJ, Brady MF, et al. Cyclophosphamide and cisplatin compared with paclitaxel and cisplatin in patients with stage III and stage IV ovarian cancer. N Engl J Med 1996; 334:1–6.
11. Vasey PA. Survival and longer-term toxicity of the SCOTROC study: docetaxel-carboplatin (DC) vs. paclitaxel-carboplatin (PC) in ovarian cancer (abstract). Proc Am Soc Clin Oncol 2002; 21:202a.
12. Shah IA, Jayram L, Gani OS, et al. Papillary serous carcinoma of the peritoneum in a man: a case report. Cancer 1998; 82:860–866.
13. Bhatia SK, Saclarides TJ, Witt TR, et al. Hormone receptor studies in axillary metastases from occult breast cancers. Cancer 1987; 59:1170–1172.
14. Block EF, Meyer MA. Positron emission tomography in diagnosis of occult adenocarcinoma of the breast. Am Surg 1998; 64:906–908.
15. Schorn C, Fisher U, Luftner-Nagel S, et al. MRI of the breast in patients with metastatic disease of unknown primary. Eur Radiol 1999; 9:470–473.
16. Rades D, Kuhnel G, Wildfang I, et al. Localised disease in cancer of unknown primary (CUP): the value of positron emission tomography (PET) for individual therapeutic management. Ann Oncol 2001; 12:1605.
17. Nguyen LN, Maor MH, Oswald MJ. Brain metastases as the only manifestation of an undetected primary tumor. Cancer 1998; 83:2181.
18. Salvati M, Cervoni L, Raco A. Single brain metastases from unknown primary malignancies in CT-era. J Neurooncol 1995; 23:75.
19. Motzer RJ, Rodriguez E, Reuter VE, et al. Molecular and cytogenetic studies in the diagnosis of patients with midline carcinomas of unknown primary site. J Clin Oncol 1995; 13:274–282.
20. Williams SD, Birch R, Einhorn LH, et al. Treatment of disseminated germ cell tumors with cisplatin, bleomycin, and either vinblastine or etoposide. N Engl J Med 1987; 316:1435–1440.

21. Fox RM, Woods RL, Tattersall MHN. Undifferentiated carcinoma in young men: the atypical teratoma syndrome. Lancet 1979; 1:1316–1318.
22. Greco FA, Vaughn WK, Hainsworth JD. Advanced poorly differentiated carcinoma of unknown primary site: recognition of a treatable syndrome. Ann Intern Med 1986; 104:547–553.
23. Hainsworth JD, Greco FA. Poorly differentiated carcinoma of unknown primary site. In: Fer MF, Greco FA, Oldham R, eds. Poorly Differentiated Neoplasms and Tumors of Unknown Origin. Orlando, FL: Grune and Stratton, 1986:189–202.
24. Richardson RL, Schoumacher RA, Fer MF, et al. The unrecognized extragonadal germ cell cancer syndrome. Ann Intern Med 1981; 94:181–186.
25. Hainsworth JD, Johnson DH, Greco FA. Cisplatin-based combination chemotherapy in the treatment of poorly differentiated carcinoma and poorly differentiated adenocarcinoma of unknown primary site: results of a 12-year experience. J Clin Oncol 1992; 10:912–922.
26. Jones AS, Cook JA, Phillips DE, Roland NR. Squamous carcinoma presenting as an enlarged cervical lymph node. Cancer 1993; 72:1756–1761.
27. Carlson LS, Fletcher GH, Oswald MJ. Guidelines for the radiotherapeutic techniques for cervical metastases from an unknown primary. Int J Radiat Oncol Biol Phys 1986; 12:2101–2110.
28. Reddy SP, Marks JE. Metastatic carcinoma in the cervical lymph nodes from an unknown primary site: results of bilateral neck plus mucosal irradiation vs ipsilateral neck irradiation. Int J Radiat Oncol Biol Phys 1997; 37:797–802.
29. Spiro RH, DeRose G, Strong EW. Cervical node metastasis of occult origin. Am J Surg 1983; 146:441–446.
30. Yang ZY, Hu YH, Yan JH, et al. Lymph node metastases in the neck from an unknown primary. Report on 113 patients. Acta Radiol Oncol 1983; 22:17–22.
31. Grau C, Johansen LV, Jakobsen J, et al. Results from a national survey by the Danish Society for Head and Neck Oncology. Radiother Oncol 2000; 55:121–129.
32. de Braud F, Heilbrun LK, Ahmed K, et al. Metastatic squamous cell carcinoma of an unknown primary localized to the neck. Advantages of an aggressive treatment. Cancer 1989; 64:510–515.
33. Jeremic B, Zivic L, Jevremovic S. Radiotherapy and cisplatin in metastatic squamous cell carcinoma of an unknown primary tumor localized to the neck. A phase II study. J Chemother 1992; 4:399–402.
34. Guarischi A, Keane TJ, Elhakim T. Metastatic inguinal nodes from an unknown primary neoplasm. A review of 56 cases. Cancer 1987; 59:572–577.
35. Hainsworth JD, Greco FA. Neoplasms of unknown primary site. In: Kufe DW, Pollock RE, et al. eds. Cancer Medicine. 6th ed. Hamilton: BC Decker, Inc., 2003:2277–2290.
36. Kasimis BS, Wuerker RB, Malefatto JP, Moran EM. Prolonged survival of patients with extrapulmonary small cell carcinoma arising in the neck. Med Pediatr Oncol 1983; 11:27–30.
37. van der Gaast A, Verweij J, Prins E, Splinter TAW. Chemotherapy as treatment of choice in extrapulmonary undifferentiated small cell carcinomas. Cancer 1990; 65:422–424.

38. McKay CE, Hainsworth JD, Burris HA, et al. Treatment of metastatic poorly differentiated neuroendocrine carcinoma with paclitaxel/carboplatin/etoposide (PCE): a Minnie Pearl Cancer Research Network phase II trial (abstract). Proc Am Soc Clin Oncol 2002; 21:158a.

39. Moertel CG, Evols LF, O'Connell MJ, Rubin J. Treatment of neuroendocrine carcinomas with etoposide and cisplatin: evidence of major therapeutic activity in anaplastic variants of these neoplasms. Cancer 1991; 68:227–232.

40. Greco FA, Thomas M, Hainsworth JD. Poorly differentiated carcinoma (PDC) or adenocarcinoma (PDA) of unknown primary site: long-term follow-up after cisplatin-based chemotherapy (abstract). Proc Am Soc Clin Oncol 1997; 16:274a.

41. Currow DC, Findlay M, Cox K, Harnett PR. Elevated germ cell markers in carcinoma of uncertain primary site do not predict response to platinum based chemotherapy. Eur J Cancer 1996; 32A:2357–2359.

42. Lenzi R, Hess KR, Abbruzzese MC, et al. Poorly differentiated carcinoma and poorly differentiated adenocarcinoma of unknown origin: favorable subsets of patients with unknown primary carcinoma? J Clin Oncol 1997; 15:2056–2062.

43. Saghatchian M, Fizazi K, Borel C, et al. Carcinoma of unknown primary site: a chemotherapy strategy based on histological differentiation–results of a prospective study. Ann Oncol 2001; 12:535–540.

8

Chemotherapy for Patients with Metastatic Carcinoma of Unknown Primary Site

F. Anthony Greco
Sarah Cannon Research Institute, Nashville, Tennessee, U.S.A.

Stéphane Culine
Centre Val d'Aurelle, Montpellier, France

INTRODUCTION

The literature regarding chemotherapy for patients with unknown primary cancers is relatively scant and requires interpretation in light of the many limitations of the available data. These patients represent an extremely heterogeneous population with respect to age, clinical presentation, sites of metastasis, functional status, and histology. Difficulties in classification has limited cooperative group studies and only in the last several years have a few investigators performed prospective therapeutic trials in groups of these patients. Treatment has improved for many specific subsets of these patients as our knowledge has continued to evolve, with an increasing ability to separate groups with important therapeutic implications. The details of the various clinical and pathological subsets of patients, which have now been fairly well characterized, have been summarized elsewhere (1,2). The classification and further deliniation of various groups also continues to evolve and is likely to expand considerably with the use of molecular techniques such as gene expression profiling. Unfortunately, most patients with well-differentiated or moderately differentiated adenocarcinoma and poorly differentiated carcinomas of unknown primary site do not correspond or fit into one of the several favorable prognostic clinical or pathological subgroups.

HISTORICAL BACKGROUND

Various chemotherapy has produced low response rates, very few complete responses, and even fewer long-term survivals in the past. Unfortunately, most of these efforts were relatively futile. The results in several reported series of patients in 45 trials (1518 patients) reported from 1964 to 2002 (1,2) are summarized briefly as follows.

5-Fluorouracil (5-FU) was the only single agent adequately studied in previously untreated patients and the response rates ranged from 0% to 16%. Cisplatin was reported as a single agent in only one series (3) with a response rate of 19%. Single agent activity of methotrexate, doxorubicin, mitomycin-c, vincristine, and semustine have been reported in 6% to 16% (4). 5-FU, combined with doxorubicin and mitomycin-c and various modifications, have been used often, based on the demonstrated activity of these combination regimens in some gastrointestinal cancers (5–16). The combination of 5-FU and leucovorin has been inadequately evaluated, but appears relatively inactive in liver metastasis with an unknown primary (17), a group of patients often suspected of harboring gastrointestinal primaries. Response rates from a review of all these prospective clinical trials (1,2) varied from 8% to 57% (mean = 24%), complete responders less than 1%, median survival ranged from 4 to 16 months (mean = 6 months), survival at one and two years were rarely reported, and disease-free survival beyond two years was not reported.

In the last decade of the 20th century, several cisplatin-based combination chemotherapy regimens have been reported (1,2). In two small randomized comparisons (5,8) of doxorubicin, with or without cisplatin, there was no difference in median survival, but more toxicity occurred in the cisplatin-containing arms. Later, a third small randomized trial (18) showed cisplatin, epirubicin, and mitomycin-c to be superior to mitomycin-c alone (median survival 9.4 vs. 5.4 months).

All these chemotherapy trial data need to be viewed with several factors in mind. Most of these series of patients are small, and large randomized comparisons are lacking. Patients were not standardly evaluated or compared in reference to sites of metastasis (nodal vs. visceral), performance status, sex, and age. Many of the known clinical and pathological subsets associated with better responses and survival with specific treatments were not yet known.

New chemotherapy used in recent studies has improved considerably for patients with adenocarcinoma and poorly differentiated carcinoma who otherwise cannot be classified into a more treatable or favorable subset. Several new drugs with rather broad spectrum antineoplastic activity are changing the standard treatment for patients with several common epithelial cancers. These drugs include the taxanes, gemcitabine (GC), irinotecan (IC), topotecan, and vinorelbine.

THE MINNIE PEARL CANCER RESEARCH NETWORK EXPERIENCE

The Minnie Pearl Cancer Research Network, a large community-based cooperative group, has completed five sequential prospective phase II trials incorporating paclitaxel (19,20), docetaxel (20,21), GC (22), and IC (23) into the first-line therapy for 396 patients with carcinoma of unknown primary site since 1995. Patients with carcinoma of unknown primary site (any histology) who were not defined in a "treatable" or favorable subset were entered in these trials (with the exception of eight patients with poorly differentiated neuroendocrine carcinoma on the first two trials). The chemotherapy protocols, patient characteristics, response rates, and survivals are summarized in Tables 1 and 2. The total response rate for all patients was 30% (107 of 353 evaluable patients), with 85 (94%) partial responders and 22 (6%) complete responders. The median survival is 9.1 months, and the one-, two-, three-, five-, and eight-year survivals are 38%, 19%, 12%, 8%, and 6%, respectively (Fig. 1). The median progression-free survival is five months, and the one-, two-, three-, five-, and eight-year progression-free survivals are 17%, 7%, 5%, 4%, and 3%, respectively (Fig. 2). The toxicity of all these regimens was primarily myelosuppression, usually moderate, with a total of eight (2%) treatment-related deaths.

The long-term follow-up on the first 144 patients (trials 1, 2, 3) is as follows: With a minimum follow-up of 4.8 years (range 4.8–8 years); the median survival is 10 months, and the one-, two-, three-, five-, and eight-year survivals are 42%, 22%, 18%, 12%, and 10%, respectively. The actuarial survival curves are similar for the 252 additional patients treated in trials 4 and 5. There is no difference in survival in any of the studies. The effectiveness of new therapy should be based on the survival and progression-free survival at one year and beyond, as there are more important milestones than median survival alone. There was no difference in survival for poorly differentiated carcinomas versus adenocarcinoma. Women survived longer than men, and those with performance status 0 and 1 [Eastern Cooperation Oncology Group (ECOG) scale] lived longer than those with performance status 2.

THE FRENCH EXPERIENCE

Several strategies of chemotherapy in both monocentric and muticenter prospective trials were explored: high-dose chemotherapy with hematopoietic stem cell support (24), dose-dense chemotherapy with hematopoietic growth factor support (25), chemotherapy based on histological differentiation (26),

Table 1 Chemotherapy Regimens and Patient Characteristics of Five Consecutive Prospective Phase II Studies in 396 Patients from 1995–2002 by the Minnie Pearl Cancer Research Network

Characteristics	Study 1[a] (19)	Study 2[b] (21)	Study 3[c] (21)	Study 4[d] (22)	Study 5[e] (23)	Total
Number of patients	71	26	47	120	132	396
Age (yrs)						
Median	72	60	56	58	59	62
Range	31–82	34–74	23–76	21–85	29–83	21–85
Male/female	35/36	13/13	25/22	64/56	67/65	203/193
Histology						
Adenocarcinoma (well-differentiated)	34 (48%)	13 (50%)	18 (38%)	63 (53%)	59 (44%)	187 (47%)
PDC or PDA	30 (42%)	11 (43%)	28 (60%)	56 (46%)	72 (55%)	197 (50%)
Neuroendocrine carcinoma (poorly differentiated)	6 (9%)	2 (7%)	0 (0%)	0 (0%)	0 (0%)	8 (2%)
Squamous carcinoma	1 (1%)	0 (0%)	1 (2%)	1 (1%)	1 (1%)	4 (1%)
ECOG performance status						
0	9 (13%)	10 (38%)	9 (19%)	27 (27%)	24 (18%)	79 (20%)
1	50 (70%)	10 (38%)	26 (55%)	77 (64%)	97 (73%)	260 (66%)
2	12 (17%)	6 (24%)	12 (26%)	16 (14%)	11 (9%)	57 (14%)
Number of organ sites involved						
1	28 (39%)	7 (27%)	15 (32%)	42 (35%)	41 (31%)	133 (34%)
≥2	43 (61%)	19 (73%)	32 (68%)	78 (65%)	91 (69%)	263 (66%)

[a]Paclitaxel + carboplatin + etoposide
[b]Docetaxel + cisplatin
[c]Docetaxel + carboplatin
[d]Paclitaxel + carboplatin + GC
[e]Paclitaxel + carboplatin + etoposide followed by GC + IC
Abbreviations: PDC, poorly differentiated carcinoma; PDA, poorly differentiated adenocarcinoma; ECOG, Eastern Cooperative Oncology Group; GC, gemcitabine; IC, irinotecan.
Source: From Ref. 40.

Table 2 Response to Therapy and Survival of Patients in the Minnie Pearl Cancer Research Network Experience

	Study 1	Study 2	Study 3	Study 4	Study 5	Total
Number of patients	71	26	47	120	132	396
Partial response/	48%/	22%/	22%/	21%/	23%/	30%/
complete response	15%	4%	0%	4%	6%	6%
1-year survival	48%	40%	33%	42%	35%	38%
2-year survival	20%	28%	28%	23%	16%	19%
3-year survival	14%	16%	15%	14%	Too early	12%
5-year survival	12%	13%	10%	Too early	Too early	10%
8-year survival	8%	Too early	Too early	Too early	Too early	8%
Minimum follow-up (yr)	6.7	6	4.8	3	1	1
Range of follow-up (yr)	6.7–8	6–6.7	4.8–5.8	3–4.6	1–2	1–8

Source: From Ref. 40.

and screening of new regimens, namely, cisplatin in combination with GC or IC (27) or GC combined with docetaxel (28).

At the Montpellier Cancer Center, a prospective high-dose intensity policy was developed from June 1995 to December 1999 with survival as primary endpoint. In 20 patients with age less than 61 years, ECOG performance status of 0 or 1, poorly differentiated adenocarcinoma or poorly differentiated carcinoma, and no evidence of brain and bone marrow involvement, the treatment plan included four sequential high-dose alternative

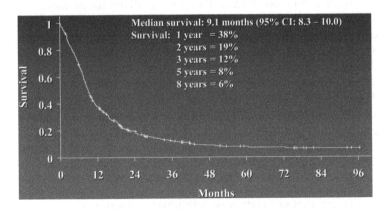

Figure 1 Unknown primary carcinoma trials: combined overall survival. Survival curve for 396 patients treated on five sequential prospective phase II trials by the Minnie Pearl Cancer Research Network. *Source*: From Ref. 40.

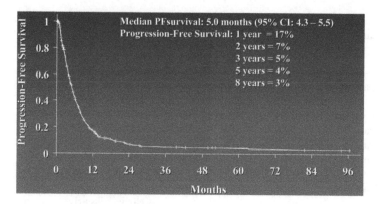

Figure 2 Unknown primary carcinoma trials: PF survival curve for 396 patients treated on five sequential prospective phase II trials by the Minnie Pearl Cancer Research Network. *Abbreviation*: PF, progression-free. *Source*: From Ref. 40.

courses combining doxorubicin/cyclophosphamide and etoposide and carboplatin with hematopoietic progenitor cell and growth factor support. In 82 other patients who did not comply with the above criteria, alternative bimonthly cycles of doxorubicin/cyclophosphamide and etoposide/cisplatin were given with granulocyte macrophage-colony stimulating factor support. The overall median survivals were 11 and 10 months, respectively (24,25). From December 2000 to April 2003, 35 patients were treated with a combination of docetaxel and GC. The median overall survival time was 10 months (28).

At Institut Gustave Roussy, Villejuif, a chemotherapy strategy based on histological differentiation was designed from 1993 to 1998. Thirty patients with poorly differentiated carcinoma or poorly differentiated adenocarcinoma received a combination of cisplatin and etoposide. Eighteen patients with well- or moderately differentiated carcinoma received cisplatin, continuous infusion of 5-FU, and alpha-interferon. Median survivals were 9 and 16 months, respectively (26).

The French Study Group on Carcinomas of Unknown Primary (GEFCAPI) conducted a randomized phase II study in 14 cancer centers from August 1999 to November 2000 with the aim of assessing the efficacy of cisplatin in combination with GC or IC. With a median follow-up of 22 months, the median survivals were 8 and 6 months in the GC and IC arms, respectively (27).

AT THE END, DOES CHEMOTHERAPY IMPROVE SURVIVAL?

Randomized prospective clinical trials proving that any form of chemotherapy improves the survival of these patients over best supportive care alone have not been reported. Nonetheless, it certainly appears survival is now better than in the past. Historical control data are associated with several difficulties, particularly the heterogeneous patient population with so many variables representing multiple subsets of patients. Prospective clinical trial survival data (1,2) are helpful, but nearly all the results report only median survivals. In some of these early trials the one-year survivals were 10% to 20%, but two-, three-, and five-year survivals were not reported probably because of early reporting or all the patients had died. Retrospective reviews can be useful, but suffer from even greater variability than prospective results.

Several reports of survival for large numbers of patients with unknown primary cancer are available for review (28–36) (Table 3) and may better define the natural history of these patients. These reviews were generally retrospective; therefore, treatments were not uniform, and some patients received local therapy or no therapy. These series also contained patients now known to fit into specific treatable or otherwise favorable subsets. Conversely, some of these patients were debilitated and near death at the time of diagnosis. There are 31,419 reported patients in these series (Table 3). The median survival was five months with a one-year survival of 22% and five-year survival of 5%. The survival at one year and beyond is largely represented by subsets of patients with a more favorable prognosis (squamous cell in neck nodes) who received local therapy (surgery or radiotherapy) or those with very indolent tumors (such as carcinoids). This conclusion is supported by data in Table 4. Squamous (epidermoid) carcinoma and well-differentiated neuroendocrine carcinoma (carcinoid, islet cell type

Table 3 Unknown Primary Cancer: Survival of All Patients[a]

Study	No. of patients	Median survival (mos)	1-Year survival (%)	5-Year survival (%)
Yale University (28)	1268	5	23	6
M.D. Anderson (29)	1000	11	43	11
University of Kansas (30)	686	6	21.5	5.1
Charity Hospital (31)	453	4	13.9	3.3
Johns Hopkins (32)	245	3	18	2
Mayo Clinic (33)	150	4	12	0.7
Southeast Netherlands (34)	1024	2.75	15	NR
Switzerland (35)	543	4	15	NR
SEER (36)	26,050	NR	NR	5
Total	31,419	5	22	5

[a]Includes treated and untreated patient groups, all histologies, and clinical presentations.
Abbreviations: SEER, Surveillance, Epidemiology, and End Results Registries; NR, not reported.
Source: From Ref. 40.

Table 4 Survival of Patients with Squamous Cell Carcinoma and Well-Differentiated Neuroendocrine Carcinoma[a]

Study: center (Reference)	Number (N)	Median survival (mos)	1-Year survival (%)	5-Year survival (%)
Squamous cell carcinoma: Yale (28)	148	9	39	15
All other patients: Yale	1120	5	21	5
Squamous cell carcinoma: M.D. Anderson (29)	62	38	85	43
Well-differentiated neuroendocrine carcinoma: M.D. Anderson	43	26	75	34
All other patients: M.D. Anderson	895	9	35	8
Squamous cell carcinoma: Switzerland (35)	48	10.1	NR	NR
All other patients: Switzerland	495	4	15	NR
Epidermoid carcinoma: SEER (36)	2670	NR	NR	30
All other patients: SEER	23,380	NR	NR	5
Total:				
Squamous/neuroendocrine	2971	20[b]	66[b,c]	30[c]
All other patients	25,890	6[b]	20[b]	5[c]

[a]Includes treated and untreated patients
[b]SEER data not included in calculation (not reported).
[c]Switzerland data not included in calculation (not reported).
Abbreviations: SEER, Surveillance, Epidemiology, and End Results Registries; NR, not reported.
Source: From Ref. 40.

histology) reported from some series (total of 2971 patients) had median, one-year and five-year survival rates of 20 months, 66% and 30%, respectively. All the remaining patients in these series (total of 25,890 patients) had median, one-year, and five-year survival rates of 6 months, 20%, and 5%, respectively.

These historical data make a very compelling and logical argument that the newer chemotherapy regimens as administered in prospective clinical trials by the Minnie Pearl Research Network to 396 patients with relatively poor prognostic features produces a meaningful prolongation of survival for these patients. The long-term survivals at one-, two-, three-, five-, and eight-years are 38%, 19%, 12%, 8%, and 6%, respectively. Survival at one year is double and at two years is similar to the one-year survival of historical control patients.

Other investigators have reported early follow-up data with the newer cytotoxic drugs including paclitaxel, docetaxel, GC, and IC-based regimens (27,28,37–39), and the median survivals are similar to the 396 patients reported here, but long-term follow-up has not yet been reported. Improvements in therapy are best seen and documented as one-, two-, three-, and five-year survival endpoints. Only about 20% of patients are long-term (greater than two years) survivors; consequently, differences in survival beyond one year may not be appreciated by comparing only median survival data.

CONCLUSION

Most patients with unknown primary adenocarcinoma or poorly differentiated carcinoma do not conform to any previously defined "treatable" or favorable subset. These patients can now attain substantial clinical benefit and prolongation of survival from the new cytotoxic drug combinations. Despite the fact that randomized trials of treatment versus no treatment have not been reported the median survival as well as one-, two-, three-, and five-year survival results are substantially superior to the survivals of these patients in the past. The survival for patients with unknown primary carcinoma now are similar to the survivals of several other groups of advanced carcinoma patients receiving various types of chemotherapy, including extensive stage small cell lung cancer and advanced nonsmall cell lung cancer. The standard therapy for good performance status patients with carcinoma of unknown primary site is with one of the newer cytotoxic combinations described above. There is major room for improvement, and basic and clinical research remains a priority in order to continue to refine and improve treatment.

REFERENCES

1. Greco FA, Hainsworth JD. Cancer of unknown primary site. In: Devita VT, Hellman S, Rosenberg SA, eds. Cancer Principles and Practice of Oncology. 6th ed. Philadelphia, Lippincott: Williams and Wilkens, 2001:2537–2560.
2. Pavlidis N, Briasoulis E, Hainsworth J, Greco FA. Diagnostic and therapeutic management of cancer of an unknown primary. Eur J Cancer 2003; 39:1990.
3. Wagener DJT, de Muelder PHM, Burghouts JT, et al. Phase II trial of cisplatin for adenocarcinoma of unknown primary site. Eur J Cancer 1991; 27:755–757.
4. Casciato DA. Metastasis of unknown origin. In: Haskell C. ed. Cancer Treatment. 4th ed. Philadelphia: W.B. Saunders Company, 1995:1128–1148.
5. Milliken ST, Tattersall MHN, Woods RL, et al. Metastatic adenocarcinoma of unknown primary site: a randomized study of two combination chemotherapy regimens. Eur J Cancer Clin Oncol 1987; 23:1645–1648.
6. McKeen E, Smith F, Haidak D, et al. Fluorouracil, adriamycin and mitomycin-C for adenocarcinoma of unknown origin [abstr]. Proc Am Assoc Cancer Res 1980; 21:358.

7. Woods RL, Fox RM, Tattersall MHN, et al. Metastatic adenocarcinoma of unknown primary: a randomized study of two combination-chemotherapy regimens. N Engl J Med 1980; 303:87–89.

8. Eagan RT, Thermean TM, Rubin J, et al. Lack of value for cisplatin added to mitomycin–doxorubicin combination chemotherapy for carcinoma of unknown primary site. Am Clin Oncol 1987; 10:82–85.

9. Goldberg RM, Smith FP, Ueno W, et al. Fluorouracil, adriamycin and mitomycin in the treatment of adenocarcinoma of unknown primary. J Clin Oncol 1986; 4:395–399.

10. Kambhu I, Kelsen D, Niedzwiecki D, et al. Phase II trial of mitomycin-C, vindesine, and adriamycin and predictive variables in the treatment of patients with adenocarcinoma of unknown primary site [abstr]. Proc Am Assoc Cancer Res 1986; 27:734.

11. Flore JJ, Kelsen DP, Gralla RJ, et al. Adenocarcinoma of unknown primary origin. Treatment with vindesine and doxorubicin. Cancer Treat Rep 1985; 69:591–594.

12. Valentine J, Rosenthal S, Arseneau JC. Combination chemotherapy for adenocarcinoma of unknown primary origin. Cancer Clin Trials 1979; 2:265–268.

13. Rudnick S, Tremont S, Staab E, et al. Evaluation and therapy of adenocarcinoma of unknown primary [abstr]. Proc Am Soc Clin Oncol 1981; 1:379.

14. Sulkes A, Uziely B, Isacson R, et al. Combination chemotherapy in metastatic tumors unknown origin. Ist J Med Sci 1988; 24:604–610.

15. Van der Gaast A, Verweij J, Planting AST, et al. 5-Fluorouracil, doxorubicin, and mitomycin c (FAM) combination chemotherapy for metastatic adenocarcinoma of unknown primary. Eur J Cancer Clin Oncol 1988; 24:765–768.

16. Treat J, Falchuk SC, Tremblay C, et al. Phase II trial of methotrexate-FAM in adenocarcinoma of unknown primary. Eur J Cancer Clin Oncol 1989; 25:1053–1055.

17. Nole F, Colleoni M, Buzzoni R, et al. Fluorouracil plus folinic acid in metastatic adenocarcinoma of unknown primary site suggestive of a gastrointestinal primary. Tumori 1993; 79:116–118.

18. Falkson CI, Cohen GL. Mitomycin-c, epirubicin and cisplatin versus mitomycin-c alone as therapy for carcinoma of unknown primary origin. Oncology 1998; 55:116.

19. Hainsworth JD, Erland JB, Kalman CA, et al. Carcinoma of unknown primary site: treatment with one-hour paclitaxel, carboplatin and extended schedule etoposide. J Clin Oncol 1997; 15:2385–2393.

20. Greco FA, Gray J, Burris HA, et al. Taxane-based chemotherapy with carcinoma of unknown primary site. Cancer J 2001; 7:203–212.

21. Greco FA, Erland JB, Morrissey LH, et al. Phase II trials with docetaxel plus cisplatin or carboplatin. Ann Oncol 2000; 11:211–215.

22. Greco FA, Burris HA, Litchy S, et al. Gemcitabine, carboplatin, and paclitaxel for patients with unknown primary site: a Minnie Pearl Cancer Research Network study. J Clin Oncol 2002; 20:1651–1656.

23. Greco FA, Hainsworth JD, Yardley DA, et al. Sequential paclitaxel/carboplatin/etoposide followed by irinotecan/gemcitabine for patients with carcinoma of unknown primary site: a Minnie Pearl Cancer Research Network phase II trial. Proc Am Soc Clin Oncol 2002; 21:161a.

24. Culine S, Fabbro M, Ychou M, et al. Chemotherapy in carcinomas of unknown primary site: a high-dose intensity policy. Ann Oncol 1999; 10:569–575.

25. Culine S, Fabbro M, Ychou M, et al. Alternative bimonthly cycles of doxorubicin, cyclophosphamide, and etoposide, cisplatin with hematopoietic growth factor support in patients with carcinoma of unknown primary site. Cancer 2002; 94:840–846.

26. Pouessel D, Culine S, Becht C, et al. Gemcitabine and docetaxel as front-line chemotherapy in patients with carcinoma of an unknown primary site. Cancer 2004; 100:1257–1261.

27. Culine S, Lortholary A, Voigt JJ, et al. Cisplatin in combination with either gemcitabine or irinotecan in carcinomas of unknown primary site: results of a randomized phase II study—trial for the French Study Group on Carcinomas of Unknown Primary (GEFCAPI 01). J Clin Oncol 2003; 21:3479–3482.

28. Altman E, Cadman E. An analysis of 1,539 patients with cancer of unknown primary site. Cancer 1986; 57:120–124.

29. Hess KR, Abbruzzese MC, Lenzi R, et al. Classification and regression free analysis of 1000 consecutive patients with unknown primary carcinoma. Clin Cancer Res 1999; 5:3403–3410.

30. Holmes FT, Fouts TL. Metastatic cancer of unknown primary site. Cancer 1970; 26:816–820.

31. Krementz ET, Cerise EJ, Foster DC, et al. Metastases of undetermined source. Curr Probl Cancer 1979; 4:1–37.

32. Markman M. Metastatic adenocarcinoma of unknown primary site: analysis of 245 patients seen at the Johns Hopkins Hospital from 1965–1979. Med Ped Oncol 1982; 10:569–574.

33. Moertel CG, Reitmeier RJ, Schutt AJ, et al. Treatment of the patient with adenocarcinoma of unknown primary site. Cancer 1972; 30:1469–1472.

34. Van de Wouw AJ, Janssen-Heijnen MLC, Coebergh JWW, et al. Epidemiology of unknown primary tumors; incidence and population-based survival of 1285 patients in Southeast Netherland 1984–1992. Eur J Cancer 2002; 38:409–413.

35. Levi F, Te VC, Erler G, et al. Epidemiology of unknown primary tumors. Eur J Cancer 2002; 38:1810–1812.

36. Muir C. Cancer of unknown primary site. Cancer 1995; 75:353.

37. Briasoulis E, Kalofonos H, Bafaloukos D, et al. Carboplatin plus paclitaxel in unknown primary carcinoma: a phase II Hellenic Cooperative Oncology Group study. J Clin Oncol 2000; 18:3101–3107.

38. Lastra E, Munoz A, Rubio I, et al. Paclitaxel, carboplatin, and oral etoposide in the treatment of patients with carcinoma of unknown primary site. Proc Am Soc Clin Oncol 2000; 19:579a.

39. Mukai H, Watanabe T, Ando M, et al. A safety and efficacy trial of docetaxel and cisplatin in patients with cancer of unknown primary. Proc Am Soc Clin Oncol 2003; 22:646.

40. Greco FA, Hainsworth JD. Cancer of unknown primary site. In: Devita VT, Hellman S, Rosenberg SA, eds. Cancer Principles and Practice of Oncology. 7th ed. Philadelphia, Lippincott: Williams and Wilkins, 2005:2213–2236.

9

Randomized Trials in Patients with Carcinoma of an Unknown Primary Site: The Past, the Present, and the Future

Karim Fizazi

Institut Gustave Roussy, Villejuif, France

Hans-Joachim Schmoll

Martin-Luther University, Halle, Germany

INTRODUCTION

Published and ongoing randomized trials in patients with carcinoma of an unknown primary site (CUP) were identified and criticized. To our knowledge, no randomized trial comparing chemotherapy versus best supportive care has been conducted in CUP to date. Seven randomized clinical trials have been published, including two randomized phase II trials. The shortcoming in all of these trials is the limited number of recruited patients, which signifies that the trials were inadequately powered to detect a small survival difference. Of the three trials that compared a cisplatin-containing regimen to another chemotherapy regimen, one reported a benefit both in terms of response and overall survival. The second trial showed a nonstatistically significant trend in overall survival in favor of the cisplatin arm. In the third trial, no difference was found, although this might be related to the low dose intensity and the short duration of cisplatin administration. Anthracycline-containing regimens apparently increased response rates in two randomized trials although the difference might also be related to another drug, given the multiplicity of agents in the different chemotherapy regimens. On the basis of the results of one randomized trial, closed early due to poor accrual, it is unlikely that mitomycin-c increases survival in CUP patients. Lastly, a phase II randomized trial showed promising activity with both the cisplatin/ gemcitabine and the cisplatin/irinotecan regimens, with different patterns of toxicity, and this was the rationale for an ongoing phase III trial.

Seven ongoing or completed, but unpublished, randomized trials were identified by the authors and are described and commented on in this chapter. A contact e-mail address and/or phone number is provided to ease and stimulate participation in these trials. Potential ideas and recommendations for future prospective randomized trials in CUP are provided in this chapter.

Randomization is currently the most accurate way to ascertain that one treatment is better than another treatment. This is why evidence-based medicine is mostly structured on the results of randomized trials.

In patients with a CUP, however, only a few randomized trials have been conducted, and they usually recruited only a limited number of patients (Tables 1 and 2). For example, although the activity of various chemotherapy regimens has been regularly demonstrated in CUP in phase II trials with response rates typically in the 20% to 50% range, a survival benefit with chemotherapy versus best supportive care has never been tested in prospective randomized trials, in contrast with other neoplasms including colorectal cancer or lung cancer. The limited number of available randomized trials makes it difficult to identify a standard treatment in patients with CUP whose disease does not fit into a specific clinico-pathological entity (see Chapters 4 and 7 for definition).

In recent years, however, many groups have advocated that randomized trials be conducted in patients with CUP (1), and more of such randomized trials have been published or initiated during the last five years than in the hitherto published literature. This is why it seemed to us worthwhile and potentially important for the oncologist to review past, present, and future randomized trials in CUP.

METHODS

We conducted a systematic search of Medline for published papers using the keywords "carcinoma," "unknown," and either "randomized" or "randomised." This was completed by data obtained from the large systematic review of the literature on CUP, recently performed by the "Standards, Options, and Recommendations" group of experts (summarized in 2, 3). All selected articles were critically reviewed and analyzed.

A search of PDQ was performed for ongoing randomized trials of CUP. To ensure that this review was as extensive as possible, it was completed by direct contact (either by phone or by email) with identified leaders in the field of CUP to determine whether they were aware of ongoing randomized trials in CUP patients.

Table 1 Completed (Published) Randomized Trials in CUP

Author, Reference (Institution)	Number of patients	Chemotherapy	Response rate %	Median PFS (mo)	Median OS (mo)
Huebner (11) (German CUP Study Group)	90	Carboplatin + paclitaxel vs. Gemcitabine + vinorelbine	21.5 21.5	6.4 4.0	10.7 6.9
Culine (9) (GEFCAPI, France)	80	Cisplatin + gemcitabine vs. Cisplatin + irinotecan	55 38	5 4	8 6
Assersohn (10) (Multicenter, United Kingdom)	88	5-FU (PVI) vs. 5-FU (PVI)+ mitomycin-c	11.6 20 (NS)	4.1 3.6 (NS)	6.6 4.7 (NS)
Dowell (8) (Vanderbilt, United States)	34	Carboplatin + etoposide vs. Paclitaxel + 5-FU + FA	19 19 (NS)	NA	6.5 8.4 (NS)
Falkson (7) (University of Pretoria, South Africa)	84	Cisplatin + epirubicin + mitomycin-c vs. Mitomycin-c	50 17	4.5 2.0 ($P=0.05$)	9.4 5.4 ($P=0.05$)
Eagan (6) (Mayo Clinic, United States)	55	Cisplatin + doxorubicin + mitomycin-c vs. Doxorubicin + mitomycin-c	27 14 (NS)	NA	4.6 5.5 (NS)
Milliken (5) (Sydney, Australia)	101	Cisplatin + vinblastine + bleomycin vs. Doxorubicin + mitomycin-c	32 42 (NS)	NA	6.2 4.5 (NS)
Woods (4)	47	Cyclophosphamide + methotrexate + 5-FU vs. Doxorubicin + mitomycin-c	5 36 ($P<0.01$)		1.7 4.5 (NS)

Abbreviations: CUP, carcinoma of an unknown primary site; mo, months; PFS, progression-free survival; OS, overall survival; NS, nonsignificant; 5-FU, 5-flurouracil; PVI, protracted venous infusion; FA, folinic acid; NA, not available.

Table 2 Completed (Unpublished) and Ongoing Randomized Trials in CUP

Institution or group (country) and name of protocol chair	Planned number of patients (trial status)	Trial design (trial name)	Patient population	Treatment
GEFCAPI (France) Karim Fizazi, MD, PhD E-mail: fizazi@igr.fr	192 (ongoing)	Phase III (GEFCAPI 02 trial)	CUP with a "good" prognosis Specific CUP entities are excluded	Arm A: cisplatin + gemcitabine Arm B: cisplatin
GEFCAPI (France) Thierry Lesimple, MD E-mail: lesimple@rennes.fnclcc.fr	150 (ongoing)	Phase II–III (GEFCAPI 03 trial)	CUP with a "poor" prognosis Specific CUP entities are excluded	Arm A: capecitabine Arm B: gemcitabine Arm C: medroxyprogesterone
NCI (U.S.A.) David P. Kelsen, MD	100 (completed)	Phase III (MSKCC-8564 NCI-T85–0205D)	CUP	Arm A: expectant observation followed by chemotherapy (Doxorubicin, mitomycin-c, vinblastine) Arm B: immediate chemotherapy (same regimen)
Christie Hospital N.H.S. Trust (United Kingdom)	398 (Stopped due to poor accrual after 21 patients were recruited)	Phase III (CHNT-VAC-VS-ECF EU-20041)	Specific CUP entities are excluded	Arm A: doxorubicin, vincristine, cyclophosphamide

Juan Valle, MD E-mail: juan.valle@christie-tr.nwest.nhs.uk Academisch Ziekenhuis Maastricht (The Netherlands) R.L. Jansen, MD E-mail: rja@sint.azm.nl	130 (completed)	Phase III (DUT-KWF-CKVO-9801 EU-98023)	Specific CUP entities are excluded	Arm B: cisplatin, epirubicin, PFI 5-FU Arm A: paclitaxel + carboplatin + etoposide Arm B: 5-FU + leucovorin
Yale Comprehensive Cancer Center (U.S.A.) James Fischer, MD, PhD E-mail: jmes.fischer@yale.edu	200 (completed)	Phase III (YALE-HIC-6611 NCI-V92–0190)	Squamous-cell head and neck CUP	Arm A: radiotherapy + mitomycin-c Arm B: radiotherapy + porfiromycin
EORTC, NCIC, RTOG (European countries, U.S.A., Canada) Vincent Gregoire, MD, PhD gregoire@rbnt.ucl.ac.be	600 (ongoing)	Phase III (EORTC-24001 CAN-NCIC-EORTC-24001, DAHANCA-EORTC-24001, EORTC-22005, RTOG-EORTC-24001)	Squamous cell carcinoma of the head and neck with no identified primary	Arm A: selective irradiation of the ipsilateral neck Arm B: extensive irradiation of the neck

Abbreviation: CUP, carcinoma of an unkown primary site.

RESULTS

The Past: Published Randomized Trials in CUP

To our knowledge, eight randomized clinical trials in CUP patients have been reported so far in the medical literature (4–11). Their results are summarized in Table 1. The number of patients was limited (maximum is 101) in all these trials, either because the number of patients was not planned a priori in the trial design (4–7), or because the planned enrollment figures could not be reached due to poor accrual (10), or because the trial design was a phase II randomized trial (8,9,11). Patients with favorable clinico-pathological CUP entities (see Chapters 4 and 7 for definition) were not included in some of these trials (7–9), whereas they were included in the remaining trials (4–6,10,11). Previous chemotherapy (excepting drugs that were used in the trial) was allowed in one trial (6), whereas this criterion was not clearly mentioned in the inclusion criteria section of two trials (4,10).

Testing the Role of Cisplatin

Three trials compared a regimen including cisplatin versus a regimen without cisplatin (5–7).

In the largest trial, investigators in Australia compared the PVB regimen, originally developed in germ-cell tumors, namely, cisplatin at a dose of $60 \, mg/m^2$, vinblastine, and bleomycin, (recycled every three weeks) to doxorubicin plus mitomycin-c, in symptomatic patients with CUP (5). The response rate was similar (30% and 39%, respectively) in the two arms, and there was a nonstatistically significant trend in overall survival in favor of the PVB arm (median: 25 vs. 18 weeks).

In another trial conducted at the Mayo Clinic, Rochester, U.S.A., 55 patients were randomized to receive the combination doxorubicin/mitomycin-c, with or without cisplatin at a dose of $60 \, mg/m^2$, one cycle every four weeks (6). However, to minimize toxicity, patients were to receive only two or three cycles of the induction regimen followed by a maintenance regimen (cyclophosphamide, doxorubicin, and methotrexate) repeated once every four to six weeks. Results showed that the response rate was almost double in the cisplatin-containing arm (26% vs. 14%), although the difference did not reach significance ($P = 0.14$). Survival was similar, with a median of about five months in both arms. Besides the small number of patients, this trial was obviously limited by a number of shortcomings including that cisplatin was given at quite a low dose ($60 \, mg/m^2$/cycle), with a low dose intensity (one cycle every four weeks), and for only two or three cycles.

Finally, investigators from the University of Pretoria, South Africa, compared mitomycin-c with or without a cisplatin/epirubicin combination in a randomized trial including 84 patients (7). The results showed an improved response rate (50% vs. 17%) and complete response rate (20% vs. 8%) and longer time to progression (median: 4.5 vs. 2 months,

$P = 0.05$), and overall survival (median: 9.4 vs. 5.4 months, $P = 0.05$) in favor of the combination arm compared to the single agent mitomycin-c arm. However, these results were undermined by the fact that the two arms were not perfectly balanced in terms of metastatic sites, with less lymph node involvement (6 vs. 13) and more liver metastases (18 vs. 12) in the single agent arm. Another limitation was that the combination arm tested the adjunction of two drugs to mitomycin-c, so that the apparent improved efficacy detected in this trial may be related to either cisplatin, epirubicin, or to both.

Thus, based on current evidence, although it is plausible (and even likely) that cisplatin improves antitumor activity and survival in patients with CUP, this still remains to be formally demonstrated.

Screening New Combination Regimens: Randomized Phase II Trials in CUP

Three randomized trials attempted to identify active regimens containing "new" anticancer drugs in patients with CUP.

The French study group on CUP (GEFCAPI) designed a two-arm randomized trial assessing the efficacy of the combination cisplatin/gemcitabine and that of cisplatin/irinotecan (9). Accrual was excellent: 80 patients were recruited in less than 18 months in this national multicenter trial (GEFCAPI 01). An independent review of pathological specimens (including immunohistochemical analysis) was performed with radiologically documented tumor response validation. Both regimens were considered active in terms of response (55% and 38%, respectively), and therefore they both fulfilled the trial hypothesis. Median overall survival was eight and six months, respectively. No statistical comparison was made between arms because the trial was not designed to compare the two regimens. Two toxicity-related deaths occurred in the cisplatin/irinotecan arm causing the authors to reduce the doses in patients accrued thereafter. None occurred in the cisplatin/gemcitabine arm. This latter regimen is currently being tested in a phase III trial conducted by the same group.

Investigators from the Vanderbilt-Ingram cancer center and a medical network in Tennessee also conducted a small ($n = 34$) randomized phase II study to assess the antitumor activity of combination carboplatin/etoposide and paclitaxel/5-fluorouracil (5-FU)/leucovorin (8). The response rate was disappointingly low (19% in both arms) and median overall survival rates were 6.5 and 8.4 months, respectively. Toxicity in the carboplatin/etoposide arm was considered too high for this regimen to be recommended in routine practice at the doses used (AUC 6 on day 1 and 100 mg/m^2/day on days 1–3, repeated every four weeks, respectively).

A German multicenter group conducted a randomized phase II study ($n = 90$) to assess the practicability of combination paclitaxel/carboplatin and gemcitabine/vinorelbine (11). Results are only available in abstract form. Both groups had a high incidence of liver involvement

(59% and 69%, respectively) indicating a high-risk population. In a preliminary analysis, both regimens yielded a 21.5% response rate. Median overall survival and median progression-free survival were 10.7 and 6.4 months with a one-year survival rate of 31% in the carboplatin/paclitaxel arm. Median overall survival and median progression-free survival were 6.9 and 4.0 months with a one-year survival rate of 22% in the gemcitabine/vinorelbine arm. A formal comparison was not done due to the phase II design.

Testing Mitomycin-c-Containing Regimens

Two studies compared a mitomycin-c-containing regimen to a regimen not containing this compound (4,10).

The very first randomized trial ever published in CUP compared the CMF regimen (cyclophosphamide, methotrexate, 5-FU), which was standard treatment in advanced breast cancer at the time with the doxorubicin/mitomycin-c regimen (4). This was a small randomized trial with only 47 patients, all of whom had cancer-related symptoms. The reasons why the trial was stopped after this level of accrual was not indicated in the article. A significantly better response rate was achieved (5% vs. 36%, respectively; $P < 0.01$) and a nonstatistically significant trend towards improved median survival (4.5 vs. 1.7 months) in favor of the doxorubicin/mitomycin-c regimen. The response rate yielded by this latter regimen was subsequently confirmed by the same group in a separate set of 16 patients. Thus, two trials including this one (4,7) suggested improved efficacy with antracycline-containing regimens, although in both cases, the apparent difference may also be attributed to another drug (cisplatin in Falkson's trial and mitomycin-c in Woods' trial).

Lastly, a multicenter phase III randomized trial conducted by a British group compared protracted intravenous 5-FU with or without mitomycin-c (10). Due to poor accrual (only 88 recruited patients over a six-year period), the study was closed early, although at initiation, the plan was to include 266 patients. There was no difference in the overall response rate, which was the primary endpoint of the trial, with respectively 12% and 20% for 5-FU alone and 5-FU combined with mitomycin-c, nor in overall survival rates (median: 6.6 and 4.7 months, respectively). Although this trial, like many others, is statistically underpowered, the results suggest that clinically relevant increased survival in patients with CUP due to mitomycin-c is unlikely.

The Present: Ongoing Randomized Trials in CUP

In this chapter, only trials specifically designed for CUP patients were selected. As can be seen in Table 2, seven ongoing or completed but unpublished trials were identified. One U.S. trial (now closed) compared immediate chemotherapy versus delayed treatment. Another French trial is comparing a chemotherapy arm versus medroxyprogesterone (given in a context of "best supportive care") in patients with poor-prognosis CUP according to the GEFCAPI classification (12). Some trials are comparing two chemotherapy regimens in patients with CUP. Specific CUP entities are generally exclusion criteria in these trials. Finally, two trials are focused on patients with squamous-cell CUP of the head and neck [one trial (now closed) compared two chemotherapy drugs plus radiotherapy, while the other compared two radiotherapy modalities].

The principal investigator of each trial and his/her Email address or phone number is mentioned in Table 2, so that he/she can be contacted in order to facilitate accrual in these clinical trials, which is recommended.

Difficulties and Problems of Past and Present Randomized Trials

The problem affecting many trials, and in particular randomized trials, is that patients with different histologies and prognostic factors are mixed and the arms are not stratified for these prognostic factors. For example, if the population in one arm is imbalanced for more advanced stage patients or for neuroendocrine tumors, the results of the trial may be difficult to interpret.

This underlines the importance of (i) excluding patients with specific entities from randomized trials (and/or conducting trials specifically for these entities) and (ii) stratifying groups by known prognostic factors (12) in randomized trials in CUP.

The Future: New Concepts in Randomized Trials in CUP

Predicting or planning the future is always a difficult task, and history has taught us that the risk of an erroneous prediction is high. However, as oncology is evolving rapidly nowadays (although, so far, CUP patients have not been very concerned by this progress), we felt it important to mention several potential ways and ideas for the design of future randomized trials in patients with CUP:

- As previously mentioned, future trials should probably take into account prognostic factors validated in CUP (12) either to select or stratify patients.
- The design of future randomized trials should in principle include a calculation of the number of patients to be accrued onto the trial so that a relevant clinical hypothesis is likely to be answered.
- As the difficulty of recruiting CUP patients onto clinical trials has often been pointed out, it is recommended that multicenter national or international intergroup trials be designed in order to answer relevant medical questions in a shorter amount of time.
- New anticancer drugs, which were shown to be active in different neoplasms (e.g., lung cancer or pancreas cancer) including those

often found at necropsy in CUP patients, are good candidates that could be tested in CUP.

- New two- or three-drug combinations could be investigated prospectively, including drugs demonstrating broad-spectrum antitumor activity in many different tumor types (e.g., gemcitabine and taxanes). However, the lack of a true "standard" chemotherapy regimen in CUP makes it difficult to determine a control arm in future phase III trials.
- A strategy whereby patients are treated with chemotherapy regimens selected according to a molecular profile (e.g., microarray signature or selected genes studied by RT–PCR) may be considered.
- A greater effort should be devoted to identifying new biological targets (e.g., tyrosine kinase or other oncogene products) that are overexpressed and biologically important in CUP, so that inhibitors (including monoclonal antibodies and small molecules) can be tested in patients with CUP. Such an effort is well underway (13,14).

REFERENCES

1. Farrugia DC, Norman AR, Nicolson MC, et al. Unknown primary carcinoma: randomised studies are needed to identify optimal treatments and their benefits. Eur J Cancer 1996; 32A(13):2256–2261.
2. Bugat R, Bataillard A, Lesimple T, et al. FNCLCC. Summary of the standards, options and recommendations for the management of patients with carcinoma of unknown primary site (2002). Br J Cancer 2003; 89(suppl 1):S59–S66. Available at www.fnclcc.fr.
3. Lesimple T, Voigt JJ, Bataillard A, et al. FNCLCC. Clinical practice guidelines: standards, options and recommendations for the diagnosis of carcinomas of unknown primary site. Bull Cancer 2003; 90:1071–1096. Available at www.fnclcc.fr.
4. Woods RL, Fox RM, Tattersall MH, Levi JA, Brodie GN. Metastatic adenocarcinomas of unknown primary site: a randomized study of two combination-chemotherapy regimens. N Engl J Med 1980; 303:87–89.
5. Milliken ST, Tattersall MH, Woods RL, et al. Metastatic adenocarcinoma of unknown primary site. A randomized study of two combination chemotherapy regimens. Eur J Cancer Clin Oncol 1987;23:1645–1648.
6. Eagan RT, Therneau TM, Rubin J, Long HJ, Schutt AJ. Lack of value for cisplatin added to mitomycin–doxorubicin combination chemotherapy for carcinoma of unknown primary site. A randomized trial. Am J Clin Oncol 1987; 10:82–85.
7. Falkson CI, Cohen GL, Mitomycin C. epirubicin and cisplatin versus mitomycin C alone as therapy for carcinoma of unknown primary origin. Oncology 1998; 55:116–121.
8. Dowell JE, Garrett AM, Shyr Y, Johnson DH, Hande KR. A randomized phase II trial in patients with carcinoma of an unknown primary site. Cancer 2001; 91:592–597.

9. Culine S, Lortholary A, Voigt JJ, et al. A Trial of the French Study Group on Carcinomas of Unknown Primary (GEFCAPI 01). Cisplatin in combination with either gemcitabine or irinotecan in carcinomas of unknown primary site: results of a randomized phase II study-trial for the French Study Group on Carcinomas of Unknown Primary (GEFCAPI 01). J Clin Oncol 2003; 21:3479–3482.

10. Assersohn L, Norman AR, Cunningham D, et al. A randomised study of protracted venous infusion of 5-fluorouracil (5-FU) with or without bolus mitomycin C (MMC) in patients with carcinoma of unknown primary. Eur J Cancer 2003; 39:1121–1128.

11. Huebner G, Steinbach S, Kohne CH, Stahl M, Kretzschmar A, Eimermacher A. Link H on behalf of the German CUP Study Group. Paclitaxel (P)/ carboplatin (C) versus gemcitabine (G)/ vinorelbine (V) in patients with adeno- or undifferentiated carcinoma of unknown primary (CUP)—a randomized prospective phase-II-trial. Proc Am Soc Clin Oncol 2005; 23:330s (Abstr 4089).

12. Culine S, Kramar A, Saghatchian M, et al. French Study Group on Carcinomas of Unknown Primary. Development and validation of a prognostic model to predict the length of survival in patients with carcinomas of an unknown primary site. J Clin Oncol 2002; 20:4679–4683.

13. Hainsworth JD, Lennington WJ, Greco FA. Overexpression of Her-2 in patients with poorly differentiated carcinoma or poorly differentiated adenocarcinoma of unknown primary site. J Clin Oncol 2000; 18:632–635.

14. Fizazi K, Voigt JJ, Lesimple T, et al. Carcinoma of unknown primary (CUP): are tyrosine kinase receptors HER-2, EGF-R, and c-KIT suitable targets for therapy? Proc Am Soc Clin Oncol 2003; 22:883.

———————————————— VI ————————————————

LOCAL TREATMENTS IN CARCINOMA OF UNKNOWN
PRIMARY SITE: IS IT RELEVANT?

———————————— **10** ————————————

Squamous Cell Carcinoma of an Unknown Primary Tumor Located in the Cervical Lymph Nodes

Marie-Christine Kaminsky
*Department of Medical Oncology, Centre Alexis Vautrin,
Vandoeuvre Les-Nancy, France*

Emmanuel Blot
Centre Henri Becquerel, Rouen, France

SUMMARY

Cervical lymph node metastases of a squamous cell carcinoma from an unknown primary tumor is a rare situation. The patient work-up includes physical examination, panendoscopy, biopsies from all suspicious sites, computed tomography (CT), and/or magnetic resonance imaging (MRI). In the absence of detectable lesions, ipsilateral tonsillectomy can discover carcinoma in about 25% of the patients. Positron emission tomography (PET) can identify primary tumors in 25% of the patients and results in a change in treatment strategy in 24% to 53% of the patients. These results still require a confirmation.

The treatment options include surgery, alone or followed by radiotherapy, and radiotherapy alone. Combined modality treatment may result in a better outcome. The extent of radiation fields remains debatable. In high-risk patients, the addition of chemotherapy seems to improve antitumor efficacy. The prognosis of patients with cervical lymph node metastases is much more favorable than that of patients with a carcinoma of an unknown primary syndrome of other localizations. Five-year survival ranges from 20% to 60%.

INTRODUCTION

The diagnosis of cervical lymph node metastases of squamous cell carcinoma from an unknown primary site is established when no primary lesion is detected by thorough physical examination, panendoscopy, and imaging. The management of this particular presentation of cancer remains a therapeutic challenge, mainly derived from head and neck squamous carcinoma treatments. The priority is given to loco-regional control. Surgery and radiation therapy are the cornerstones of the treatment.

EPIDEMIOLOGY

Cervical lymph node metastases of squamous cell carcinoma from an occult primary comprises about 2% to 5% of all patients with carcinoma of unknown primary site (1). On the other hand, node metastasis of squamous carcinoma cancer in neck lymph nodes from an unknown primary tumor comprises 2% to 4% of the total head and neck malignancies (2). The mean age ranges from 55 to 65 years in the series and the majority of patients are men (3–9). A single lymph node involvement is the most frequent clinical presentation (75% of the cases), whereas 15% of the patients have multiple ipsilateral lymph nodes and 10% have multiple bilateral lymph nodes (10,11). Metastases in the upper and middle neck are generally due to cancer of the head and neck area, whereas metastases limited to supraclavicular area are usually secondary to primaries below the clavicles (12).

PATIENT WORK-UP

The patient work-up is focused on the assessment of the histopathological diagnosis, research for a primary tumor, and the evaluation of the extent of the disease. The medical history of the patient is collected, particularly for risk factors (alcohol and tobacco use, professional exposures, and native country). The clinical aspect of the lymph nodes is unspecific. The physical examination must specify the characteristics of the lymph node, i.e., number, topography, size, consistence, limits, and mobility. It is followed by an examination of the skin, the ears, the thyroid, an inspection of all visible mucosa, a bimanual palpation of the floor of mouth, and the tongue, by a mirror examination, and/or by naso-fibroscopic examination. A total clinical examination should also be performed.

Head and neck imaging includes CT from the clavicles to the base of the skull in order to confirm the lymph nodal origin of the mass and to specify the location, extension and relationship with the vessels, arteries, and muscles (13). CT scan can detect 5% to 20% of primary tumors (14,15). Magnetic resonance is an option. In patients with multiple and/or bilateral lymph nodes, and/or a node greater than 6 cm or lower cervical lymph nodes, a chest CT scan should be performed to exclude a thoracic primary and thoracic metastases.

Patients should subsequently undergo an extended endoscopic evaluation of the head and neck cavities (oral cavity, nasopharynx, oropharynx, hypopharynx, larynx, and nasal cavity), bronchi, and esophagus under general anesthesia. Biopsies should be performed on all suspicious sites. Many authors recommend directed blind biopsies of most likely sites of potential primary lesions, including the nasopharynx, oropharynx, oral cavity, hypopharynx, and larynx on the involved node lesion side (1,16–19).

A systematic tonsillectomy for histopathological examination is also recommended by many authors, as 23% to 28% primary tumors may be detected in the tonsil (5,20–22). The highest rate for positive tonsillectomy seem to be related to patients with subdigastric, submandibular, and/or midjugular lymph nodes (5).

Fine needle aspirations for cytologic diagnosis before neck dissection is recommended. Open biopsy is proscribed because an increased risk of local recurrences and distant metastases following this procedure was suggested (23). Squamous cell carcinomas are subclassified according to the degree of differentiation: poorly, moderately, well-differentiated, or undifferentiated.

THE ROLE OF PET

PET is a promising method to identify the occult primary in patients with head and neck squamous cell carcinoma of an unknown primary. Although this procedure remains investigational, numerous studies reported the results of PET in these patients. However, these studies usually involved a small number of patients. Furthermore, the results differ when PET was studied as a part of initial investigations (6,24–28) or when PET was studied after negative initial investigations, including negative panendoscopy with or without tonsillar excision (29–31).

When compared with the results of panendoscopy, PET shows focal tracer accumulation that indicates the primary tumor site, which is further histologically confirmed by endoscopy findings in one-third (6,25,26,28) to two-third (24,27) of patients. When PET is performed after a negative panendoscopy, with or without tonsillectomy and a negative imaging, it is able to identify a primary site in less than one-third of patients (29–31). Moreover, PET shows a primary cancer located outside of the head and neck area in 12% to 50% of patients (25,27,30,31), and the findings of PET resulted in a change in treatment strategy in 24% to 53% of patients (25,27,29–31). In addition, focal tracer accumulation corresponds to false positive and/or false negative results in 12% to 50% (6,24–30,32).

In conclusion, PET seems to be a promising technique in patients with squamous cell carcinoma of cervical node from unknown primary with a negative panendoscopy, allowing recognition of the primary tumor and modification of treatment in a significant proportion of cases. These preliminary results need confirmation with further powerful studies involving large numbers of patients.

STAGING

Neoplasms may be staged according to the sixth edition of the TNM of the American Joint Committee on Cancer and the International Union Against Cancer:

1. N1: Metastasis in a single ipsilateral lymph node, 3 cm or less in greatest dimension.
2. N2: Metastasis in a single ipsilateral lymph node, more than 3 cm but not more than 6 cm in greatest dimension; or in multiple ipsilateral lymph nodes, none more than 6 cm in greatest dimension; or in bilateral or contralateral lymph nodes, none more than 6 cm in greatest dimension.

   - N2a: Metastasis in a single ipsilateral lymph node, more than 3 cm but not more than 6 cm in greatest dimension.
   - N2b: Metastasis in multiple ipsilateral lymph nodes, none more than 6 cm in greatest dimension.
   - N2c: Metastasis in bilateral or contralateral lymph nodes, none more than 6 cm in greatest dimension.

3. N3: Metastasis in a lymph node more than 6 cm in greatest dimension.

PROGNOSIS

In contrast with diffuse metastatic carcinomas of unknown primary, survival for cervical lymph node metastases of squamous cell carcinoma patients is better. Five-year survival ranges from 20% to 60% (1,33,34). Indications for treatment of cervical lymph node metastases of squamous cell carcinoma from unknown primary depends on prognostic factors and the extent of the disease.

The importance and location of node involvement are related to prognosis and survival, because primary cancer can be more frequently out of radiation fields when node involvement is in the lower part of neck (8,9,33,35–41). Some pathological findings have also been reported to be prognostic factors: extracapsular extension (3,8,36,40–42) and undifferentiated carcinoma (35). In addition, the association of both surgical and radiation therapy have been reported to be more effective in avoiding recurrences or emerging primary or new cancer (3,33,35,37,43). In a retrospective study, other factors, i.e., hemoglobin level, age, and overall duration of treatment, were also reported to be prognostic factors for survival (9). These results argue first for a surgical excision, which can also provide pathological information and second for an intensive treatment by adding radiation therapy to surgical excision.

TREATMENT

To our knowledge, no controlled study has been published about the treatment of cervical lymph node metastases of squamous cell carcinoma from an unknown primary. Only retrospective, single-institution studies reported the results of treatment in these patients. As a consequence, when investigations for primary cancer or other metastatic site are negative, treatment with curative intent derives from head and neck cancer treatment procedures (9). Some studies also showed that primary head and neck squamous cell carcinoma could arise during the follow-up in 3% to 20% of patients with lymph node metastases of squamous cell carcinoma from unknown primary (36,44).

Surgery

In cervical metastases of squamous cell carcinoma of unknown primary, node excision can be necessary for diagnosis. Neck dissection of the involved cervical side should be the standard procedure for surgical treatment for these patients, except for supraclavicular node metastasis or cervical involvement that cannot be removed by surgical excision. Indeed, the number of involved nodes and some pathological findings can influence treatment strategy. Moreover, adenectomy could underevaluate the extent of nodal disease. As discussed in the diagnosis section, bilateral tonsillectomy has been reported to improve prognosis in these patients (22), but this effect was not reported in all the series.

Surgical excision as the sole treatment could be discussed in a few cases, mainly when the involved node is unique. However, some reports showed a worse loco-regional control when surgical excision is not followed by radiation therapy in comparison to the association of surgery and radiotherapy (33,35,37,43).

Radiation Therapy

Radiation therapy following surgical excision has been reported to improve the risk of local-regional relapse (8,9,36,40,45,46) and survival (3,8,40). As a consequence, postoperative radiotherapy is usually reported to be the standard treatment after neck excision in these patients. The dose of radiation is decided with regards to pathological examination, from 50 Gy when excision is complete to 70 Gy when pathological findings are unfavorable, i.e., showing extranodal spread, positive resection margins, perineural involvement, or vascular tumor embolism.

Radiation therapy as the sole treatment may be discussed in a few cases, mainly for a unique CT-confirmed involved node or for patients with a poor performance status and who do not allow surgical treatment. These patients are usually not able to receive chemotherapy associated with radiation treatment. Nevertheless, it seems difficult to treat such patients without node pathological examination, and the morbidity of a neck dissection versus an adenectomy alone seems to be light. Therefore, neck dissection should be proposed to patients with N1 stage, even if it was not demonstrated to improve survival or local-regional control (35).

Another question to be raised in patients receiving postoperative radiotherapy is the extent of radiation fields. Some studies reported a survival benefit of extended radiation fields (bilateral neck and mucosal irradiation) because of a reduced number of loco-regional relapses (9,36) and/or a reduced number of head and neck cancers arising during survival (36), which is often considered as the initial unknown primary. Indeed, extended fields can have a potential effect on a microscopic primary cancer (37), but increase notably the toxicity of radiation treatment (33). In fact, this question will be solved when the results of a randomized study from the European Organization for Research and Treatment of Cancer (and other groups) become available. This study compares selective radiotherapy (ipsilateral neck node area) versus extensive radiotherapy (naso, oro, hypopharyngeal, and laryngeal mucosa and neck node areas on both sides) after neck excision for squamous cell carcinoma from unknown primary.

Chemotherapy

The interest of adding chemotherapy to radiation therapy has not been investigated in this subset of patients, but it was demonstrated to be suitable (47). When neck dissection has not been performed because of major neck involvement, and with regard to head and neck cancers usual treatment (48–50), platin-containing regimen of chemotherapy could be added to radiation therapy (3).

Moreover, in poor prognosis head and neck squamous cell carcinomas, adding chemotherapy to postoperative radiation treatment improves loco-regional control (51,52) and probably survival (51). Therefore, in cervical node involvement of squamous cell carcinoma of unknown origin, irradiation with concomitant chemotherapy (cisplatin $100\,mg/m^2$ on days 1, 22, and 43 of the radiotherapy regimen) should be considered, with regards to increased acute toxicity, when clinical (N2 or N3) or pathological findings (i.e., extranodal spread or positive resection margins, perineural involvement or vascular tumor embolism) indicate unfavorable prognosis (53).

FOLLOW-UP

Several authors recommend a regular follow-up, consisting of a clinical examination and a nasofibroscopy every three months during the first two years, then every six months the next three years, then an annual examination. A chest radiograph can be performed every year. Thyroid function must be tested in patients who received neck irradiation.

During the follow-up, 10% to 20% of the patients develop a subsequent primary lesion i.e., head and neck, lung, esophagus and others, mainly during the first two years (16,54–57). An occult primary may become clinically detectable after a variable time interval, but this occurrence is rather rare and becomes exceptional when irradiation radiation therapy has been delivered on the neck after surgical excision (58). Prognosis for patient with a primary tumor occurring after initial treatment is usually poor (16,59).

REFERENCES

1. Jereczek-Fossa BA, Jassem J, Orecchia R. Cervical lymph node metastases of squamous cell carcinoma from an unknown primary. Cancer Treat Rev 2004; 30:153–164.
2. Million RR, Cassisi NJ, Manguso AA. The unknown primary. In: Management of Head and Neck Cancer: A Multidisciplinary Approach. 2d ed. Philadelphia: JB Lippincott, 1999:311–320.
3. Strojan P, Anicin A. Combined surgery and postoperative radiotherapy for cervical lymph node metastases from an unknown primary tumor. Radiother Onkol 1998; 49:33–40.
4. Oen AL, De Boer MF, Hop WC, Knecht P. Cervical metastasis from unknown primary tumor. Eur Arch Otolaryngol 1995; 252:222–228.
5. Lapeyre M, Malissard L, Peiffert D, Hoffstetter S, Toussaint B, Renier S. Cervical lymph node metastasis from an unknown primary: is a tonsillectomy necessary? Int J Radiat Oncol Biol Phys 1997; 39:292–296.
6. Mendenhall WM, Mancuso AA, Parsons JT, Stringer SP, Casisi NJ. Diagnosis evaluation of squamous cell carcinoma metastatic to cervical lymph nodes from an unknown head and neck primary site. Head Neck 1998; 20:2739–2744.
7. Berker JL, Zhen WK, Hoffmann HT, McCuloch TM, Buatti JM. Squamous cell carcinoma metastatic to cervical lymph nodes from unknown primary: a changing disease. Int J Radiat Oncol Biol Phys 2000; 48:320.
8. Colletier PJ, Garden AS, Morrison WH, Goepfert H, Geara F, Aug KK. Postoperative radiation for squamous cell carcinoma metastatic to cervical lymph nodes from an unknown primary site: outcomes and patterns of failure. Head Neck 1998; 20:674–681.
9. Grau C, Johansen LV, Jakobsen J, Geertsen P, Andersen E, Jensen BB. Cervical lymph node metastases from unknown primary tumours. Results from a national survey by the Danish Society for Head and Neck Oncology. Radiother Oncol 2000; 55:121–129.
10. Erkal HS, Mendenhall WM, Amdur RJ, Villaret DB, Stringer SP. Squamous cell carcinomas metastatic to cervical lymph nodes from an unknown head-and-neck mucosal site treated with radiation therapy alone or in combination with neck dissection. Int J Radiat Oncol Biol Phys 2001; 50:55–63.

11. Sinnathamby K, Peters LJ, Laidlaw C, Hughes PG. The occult head and neck primary: to treat or not to treat? Clin Oncol 1997; 9:322–329.
12. Barbara A, Jereczek-Fossa BA, Jassem J, Orecchia R. Cervical lymph node metastases of squamous cell carcinoma from an unknown primary. Cancer Treatment Rev 2004; 30:153–164.
13. Fitzpatrick PJ, Kotalik JF. Cervical metastases from an unknown primary tumor. Radiology 1974; 110:659–663.
14. Mancuso AA, Maceri D, Rice D, Hanafee W. CT of cervical lymph node cancer. Am J Roentgenol 1981; 136:381–385.
15. Muraki AS, Mancuso AA, Harnsberger HR. Metastatic cervical adenopathy from tumors of unknown origin: the role of CT. Radiology 1984; 152:749–753.
16. Jesse R, Perez C, Fletcher G. Cervical lymph node metastasis: unknown primary cancer. Cancer 1973; 31:854–859.
17. De Braud F, Al Sarraf M. Diagnosis and management of squamous cell carcinoma of unknown primary tumor site of the neck. Semin Oncol 1993; 20:273–278.
18. Califano J, Westra WH, Koch W, et al. Unknown primary head and neck squamous cell carcinoma: molecular identification of the site of origin. J Natl Cancer Inst 1999; 7:599–604.
19. Gabalski EC, Belles W. Management of the unknown primary in patients with metastatic cancer of the head and neck. Ear Nose Throat J 2000; 79:306–308.
20. Becuwe B, Volant A, Danie C, Leroy JP. Intérêt de l'amygdalectomie dans le bilan étiologique d'une adénopathie cervicale métastatique d'aspect kystique, et en apparence primitive. Les cahiers d'ORL 1982; 17:151–157.
21. Koch WM, Bhatti N, Williams MF, Eisele DW. Oncologic rationale for bilateral tonsillectomy in head and neck squamous cell carcinoma of unknown primary source. Otolaryngol Head Neck Surg 2001; 124:331–333.
22. Randall DA, Johnstone PA, Foss RD, Martin PJ. Tonsillectomy in diagnosis of the unknown primary tumor of the head and neck. Otolaryngol Head Neck Surg 2000; 122:52–55.
23. Robbins KT, Cole R, Marvel J, Fields R, Wolf P, Goepert H. The violated neck: cervical node biopsy prior to definitive treatment. Otolaryngol Head Neck Surg 1986; 94:605–610.
24. Stoeckli SJ, Mosna-Firlejczyk K, Goerres GW. Lymph node metastasis of squamous cell carcinoma from an unknown primary: impact of positron emission tomography. Eur J Nucl Med Mol Imag 2003; 30:411–416.
25. Bohuslavizki KH, Klutmann S, Sonnemann U, et al. F-18 FDG PET for detection of occult primary tumor in patients with lymphatic metastases of the neck region [article in German]. Laryngorhinootologie 1999; 78:445–449.
26. Greven KM, Keyes JW Jr, Williams DW III, McGuirt WF, Joyce WT III. Occult primary tumors of the head and neck: lack of benefit from positron emission tomography imaging with 2-[F-18]fluoro-2-deoxy-d-glucose. Cancer 1999; 86:114–118.
27. Assar OS, Fischbein NJ, Caputo GR, et al. Metastatic head and neck cancer: role and usefulness of FDG PET in locating occult primary tumors. Radiology 1999; 210:177–181.
28. Mukherji SK, Drane WE, Mancuso AA, Parsons JT, Mendenhall WM, Stringer S. Occult primary tumors of the head and neck: detection with 2-[F-18] fluoro-2-deoxy-D-glucose SPECT. Radiology 1996; 199:761–766.

29. Wong WL, Saunders M. The impact of FDG PET on the management of occult primary head and neck tumours. Clin Oncol (R Coll Radiol) 2003; 15: 461–466.
30. Johansen J, Eigtved A, Buchwald C, Theilgaard SA, Hansen HS. Implication of 18F-fluoro-2-deoxy-d-glucose positron emission tomography on management of carcinoma of unknown primary in the head and neck: a Danish cohort study. Laryngoscope 2002; 112:2009–2014.
31. Jungehulsing M, Scheidhauer K, Damm M, et al. 2[F]-fluoro-2-deoxy-d-glucose positron emission tomography is a sensitive tool for the detection of occult primary cancer (carcinoma of unknown primary syndrome) with head and neck lymph node manifestation. Otolaryngol Head Neck Surg 2000; 123: 294–301.
32. Perie S, Talbot JN, Monceaux G, et al. Use of a coincidence gamma camera to detect primary tumor with 18fluoro-2-deoxy-glucose in cervical lymph node metastases from an unknown origin. Ann Otol Rhinol Laryngol 2000; 109: 755–760.
33. Nieder C, Ang KK. Cervical lymph node metastases from occult squamous cell carcinoma. Curr Treat Options Oncol 2002; 3:33–40.
34. Pavlidis N, Briasoulis E, Hainsworth J, Greco FA. Diagnosic and therapeutic management of cancer of an unknown primary. Eur J Cancer 2003; 39: 1990–2005.
35. Tong CC, Luk MY, Chow SM, Ngan KC, Lau WH. Cervical nodal metastases from occult primary: undifferentiated carcinoma versus squamous cell carcinoma. Head Neck 2002; 24:361–369.
36. Iganej S, Kagan R, Anderson P, et al. Metastatic squamous cell carcinoma of the neck from an unknown primary: management options and patterns of relapse. Head Neck 2002; 24:236–246.
37. Mendenhall WM, Mancuso AA, Amdur RJ, Stringer SP, Villaret DB, Cassisi NJ. Squamous cell carcinoma metastatic to the neck from an unknown head and neck primary site. Am J Otolaryngol 2001; 22:261–267.
38. Werner JA, Dunne AA. Value of neck dissection in patients with squamous cell carcinoma of unknown primary. Onkologie 2001; 24:16–20.
39. Fernandez JA, Suarez C, Martinez JA, Llorente JL, Rodrigo JP, Alvarez JC. Metastatic squamous cell carcinoma in cervical lymph nodes from an unknown primary tumour: prognostic factors. Clin Otolaryngol 1998; 23:158–163.
40. Medini E, Medini AM, Lee CK, Gapany M, Levitt SH. The management of metastatic squamous cell carcinoma in cervical lymph nodes from an unknown primary. Am J Clin Oncol 1998; 21:121–125.
41. Maulard C, Housset M, Brunel P, et al. Postoperative radiation therapy for cervical lymph node metastases from an occult squamous cell carcinoma. Laryngoscope 1992; 102:884–890.
42. Coster JR, Foote RL, Olsen KD, Jack SM, Schaid DJ, DeSanto LW. Cervical nodal metastasis of squamous cell carcinoma of unknown origin: indications for withholding radiation therapy. Int J Radiat Oncol Biol Phys 1992; 23:743–749.
43. Yalin Y, Pingzhang T, Smith GI, Ilankovan V. Management and outcome of cervical lymph node metastases of unknown primary sites: a retrospective study. Br J Oral Maxillofac Surg 2002; 40:484–487.

44. Issing WJ, Taleban B, Tauber S. Diagnosis and management of carcinoma of unknown primary in the head and neck. Eur Arch Otorhinolaryngol 2003; 260:436–443.

45. Davidson BJ, Spiro RH, Patel S, Patel K, Shah JP. Cervical metastases of occult origin: the impact of combined modality therapy. Am J Surg 1994; 168:395–399.

46. Reddy SP, Marks JE. Metastatic carcinoma in the cervical lymph nodes from an unknown primary site: results of bilateral neck plus mucosal irradiation vs. ipsilateral neck irradiation. Int J Radiat Oncol Biol Phys 1997; 37:797–802.

47. Jeremic B, Zivic L, Jevremovic S. Radiotherapy and cisplatin in metastatic squamous cell carcinoma of an unknown primary tumor localized to the neck. A phase II study. J Chemother 1992; 4:399–402.

48. Adelstein DJ, Li Y, Adams GL, et al. An intergroup phase III comparison of standard radiation therapy and two schedules of concurrent chemoradiotherapy in patients with unresectable squamous cell head and neck cancer. J Clin Oncol 2003; 21:92–98.

49. Calais G, Alfonsi M, Bardet E, et al. Randomized trial of radiation therapy versus concomitant chemotherapy and radiation therapy for advanced-stage oropharynx carcinoma. J Natl Cancer Inst 1999; 91:2081–2086.

50. Pignon JP, Bourhis J, Domenge C, Designe L. Chemotherapy added to locoregional treatment for head and neck squamous-cell carcinoma: three meta-analyses of updated individual data. MACH-NC Collaborative Group. Meta-Analysis of Chemotherapy on Head and Neck Cancer. Lancet 2000; 355:949–955.

51. Bernier J, Domenge C, Ozsahin M, et al. European Organization for Research and Treatment of Cancer Trial 22931. Postoperative irradiation with or without concomitant chemotherapy for locally advanced head and neck cancer. N Engl J Med 2004; 350:1945–1952.

52. Cooper JS, Pajak TF, Forastiere AA, et al. Radiation Therapy Oncology Group 9501/Intergroup. Postoperative concurrent radiotherapy and chemotherapy for high-risk squamous-cell carcinoma of the head and neck. N Engl J Med 2004; 350:1937–1944.

53. Cohen EE, Lingen MW, Vokes EE. The expanding role of systemic therapy in head and neck cancer. J Clin Oncol 2004; 22:1743–1752.

54. Lefebvre JL, Coche-Dequeant B, Ton Van J, Buisset E, Adenis A. Cervical lymph nodes from an unknown primary tumor in 190 patients. Am J Surg 1990; 160:443–446.

55. Maulard C, Housset M, Brunel P, et al. Primary cervical lymph nodes of epidermoid type. Results of a series of 123 patients treated by the association surgery-radiotherapy or irradiation alone. Ann Otolaryngol Chir Cervicofac 1992; 109:6–13.

56. Spiro RH, Derose G, Strong EW. Cervical node metastasis of occult origin. Am J Surg 1983; 146:441–446.

57. Wang RC, Goepfert H, Barber AE, Wolf P. Unknown primary squamous cell carcinoma metastatic to the neck. Arch Otolaryngol Head Neck Surg 1990; 116:1388–1393.

58. Gehanno P, Veber F, Blanchet F. Metastatic cervical adenopathies appearing as primary. A propos of 124 cases. Acta Chir Belg 1983; 83:142–150.

59. Jose B, Bosch A, Caldwell WL, Frias Z. Metastasis to neck from unknown primary tumor. Acta Radiol Oncol Radiat Phys Biol 1979; 18:161–170.

11

Women with Isolated Adenocarcinoma in the Axillary Lymph Node of an Unknown Primary Site

A. Lortholary, C. El Kouri, and J. F. Ramée
Centre Catherine de Sienne, Nantes, France

P. Kerbrat
Centre Eugène Marquis, Rennes, France

INTRODUCTION

Women with isolated adenocarcinomas of axillary lymph node are a specific entity among carcinoma of unknown primary site (CUP), with a relatively good prognosis that decreases with the number of positive lymph nodes. The optimal therapeutic approaches are limited by the small number of data. The breast magnetic resonance imaging (MRI) should play an important role in the management of the local breast treatment. Recommendations of the systemic treatment (chemotherapy and/or hormonotherapy) should be the same as the treatment of breast cancer with axillary node involvement.

Females with lymph node metastases isolated to one axillary area should be suspected of having stage II breast cancer. Most patients presenting with isolated axillary lymph node metastases are females. It is in general an uncommon form of occult primary breast cancer. The differential diagnosis includes metastases from adenocarcinoma of ovary, uterus, stomach, thyroid, and kidney. The diagnosis is oriented by histopathogical examination.

Pathological evaluation could be other than adenocarcinoma; lymphoma, melanoma, or squamous cell carcinoma. When these pathological evaluations are excluded, the occult primary should be considered as an ipsilateral breast cancer (1,2).

INCIDENCE

The incidence of this uncommon presentation ranges from 0.3% to 1% of all patients with breast cancer. Among 1511 patients with CUP syndrome at the M.D. Anderson Center (1), these specific presentations do not exceed 5% of cases. Described by Halsted in 1907, the first large series of patients with axillary metastases from an unknown primary ($n = 25$) was reported in 1954 by Owen et al. (3). To date, fewer than 400 cases have been described in the literature. Two recent retrospective studies were reported by Vlastos et al. (4) among 45 patients and Blanchard and Farley among 44 women. The latter reported that 35 patients with axillary lymph node metastasis from a CUP had histological evidence of a primary carcinoma of breast cancer (5).

PRESENTATION

Median age is about 52 years (range 21–80). Usually, histopathogical examination of lymph nodes reveals an invasive ductal adenocarcinoma of grade III; Hormonal receptors (estrogen and progesterone) are negative in 70% to 80% of cases. TNM classification is often TX or To N1 MO. At diagnosis, only 5% of these patients present with distant metastases (6,7).

PARA-CLINICAL EXAMINATIONS

Isolated adenocarcinoma of axillary lymph node is defined by the presence of metastatic disease for which a primary site is undetectable on presentation. By definition, classical exploration is negative, particularly breast exploration with mammography. Breast MRI using contrast enhancement is a new imaging modality for assessing the breast. Several studies have demonstrated high (86–100%) sensitivity with this technique, but with a comparatively lower (37–97%) specificity (8–11). MRI of the breast enables the identification of an occult breast primary tumor in about 75% of women who present with adenocarcinoma in the axillary lymph nodes and can influence surgical management.

Positron emission tomography (PET) scan also can be used in the diagnosis of unknown primary carcinomas, but its value is controversial. PET using fluorine-18-fluorodeoxyglucose (FDG-PET) was able to identify the primary tumor in seven patients in a cohort of 29 patients (24%). Two of these patients with axillary lymph nodes not detected by clinical examination or mammography were identified as having breast tumor, although in this study the use of breast MRI was not reported. Moreover, the discovery of the breast tumor seems not to have altered survival (12).

TREATMENT

Because of the limited data, no optimal therapeutic approaches have been defined for this particular group of patients. The management of patients with CUP has been recently summarized by the French Study Group of Carcinomas of an Unknown Primary (GEFCAPI): Standards, Options, and Recommendations (SOR) (13). For patients with axillary lymph node involvement without primary tumor, MRI should play an important role in the management of the local breast treatment. If breast MRI does not identify a primary breast tumor, surgery and breast radiotherapy are not recommended (standard, expert agreement) (13). However, Ellerbroek et al. demonstrated an advantage of radiotherapy on the breast, in terms of local breast tumor appearance. In this series of 29 patients without mastectomy, 16 patients received radiotherapy and 13 other patients did not. At a follow-up of five years, breast cancer appeared in 57% of the patients without radiotherapy and only 17% of the patients with radiotherapy ($P = 0.06$) (14). However, this series of patients reported before breast MRI and it is not sure whether the results still apply to patients with a negative MRI.

Several studies demonstrate that breast MRI increases the proportion of patients appropriate for breast conservation treatment by identifying cancers not seen on physical examination, mammography, or ultrasound (10,15). This approach was confirmed by Vlastos et al. (4) in a study on 45 patients with a T0 N1-2 MO who received loco-regional treatment consisting of mastectomy in 29% and preservation in 71% of cases. With a follow-up of seven years, no difference was detected in locoregional recurrence (15% vs. 13%), distant metastases (31% vs. 22%), or five-year survival (75% vs. 79%) between the two groups.

Axillary lymph-node dissection is very important for the histopathological diagnosis, loco-regional control, and prognostic information (standard, expert agreement). The number of lymph node involvement is associated with survival, like nonoccult breast carcinoma. The study of the M.D. Anderson Cancer Center (4) has found that the most important determinant of survival was the number of positive nodes: five-year overall survival was 87% with one to three positive nodes compared with 42% with four or more positive nodes ($P = 0.0001$).

If the results of breast MRI are positive after surgery, radiotherapy should be proposed on the breast or postmastectomy chest and on supraclavicular area. The addition of radiotherapy had a significant impact on survival compared with patients treated with observation only (4).

In this specific entity (women with isolated adenocarcinoma of axillary lymph node), no randomized trials have been conducted on the systemic treatment of this CUP syndrome, however, recommendations should be the same as the treatment of stage II or III breast cancer. Adjuvant chemotherapy and endocrine therapy should follow the guidelines of breast cancer treatment (7).

In patients with N2 disease, neoadjuvant or preoperative chemotherapy is recommended following guidelines of breast cancer treatment (7).

PROGNOSIS

The five-year and ten-year overall survival rates are 75% and 60%, respectively (4,6,7).

CONCLUSION

The management of these patients should be identical to breast cancer patients with lymph node metastases except for the loco-regional treatment if breast MRI does not identify a primary breast cancer.

REFERENCES

1. Abbruzzese A, Abbruzzese M, Hess K, Raber M, Lenzi R, Frost P. Unknown primary carcinoma: natural history and prognostic factors in 657 consecutive patients. J Clin Oncol 1994; 12:1272–1280.
2. Hainsworth J, Greco F. Treatment of patients with cancer of an unknown primary site. N Engl J Med 1993; 329:257–263.
3. Owen HW, Dockerty MB, Gray HK. Occult carcinoma of the breast. Surg Gynecol Obstet 1954; 98:302–308.
4. Vlastos G, Jean ME, Mirza AN, et al. Feasibility of breast preservation in the treatment of occult primary carcinoma presenting with axillary metastases. Ann Surg Oncol 2001; 8:425–431.
5. Blanchard DK, Farley DR. Retrospective study of women presenting with axillary metastases from occult breast carcinoma. World J Surg 2004; 28:535–539.
6. Jackson B, Scott-Conner C, Moulder J. Axillary metastases from occult breast carcinoma: diagnosis and management. Am Surg 1995; 61:431–434.
7. Pavlidis N. Cancer of unknown primary: biological and clinical characteristics. Ann Oncol 2003; 14(suppl 3):11–18.
8. Adler DD, Wahl RL. New methods for imaging the breast: techniques, findings, and potential. Ann J Roentgenol 1995; 164:19–30.
9. Orel SG, Hochman MG, Schnall MD, Reynolds C, Sullivan DC. High-resolution MR imaging of the breast: clinical context. Radiographics 1996; 16:1385–1401.
10. Chen C, Orel SG, Harris E, Schnall MD, Czerniecki BJ, Solin LJ. Outcome after treatment of patients with mammographical magnetic resonance imaging-detected breast cancer presenting axillary lymphadenopathy. Clin Breast Cancer 2004; 5(1):72–77.
11. Harms SE, Flamig DP. MR imaging of the breast. J Magn Reson Imag 1993; 3:277–283.

12. Kole AC, Nieweg OE, Pruim J, et al. Detection of unknown occult primary tumors using positron emission tomography. Cancer 1998; 82:1160–1166.
13. Bugat R, Bataillard A, Lesimple T, et al. Summary of the standards, options and recommendations for the management of patients with carcinoma of unknown primary site (2000). Br J Cancer 2003; 89(suppl 1):59–66.
14. Ellerbroek N, Holmes F, Singletary E, Evans H, Oswald M, McNeese M. Treatment of patients with isolated axillary nodal metastases from an occult primary carcinoma consistent with breast origin. Cancer 1990; 66(7):1461–1467.
15. Olson JA, Morris EA, Van Zee KJ, Linehan DC, Borgen PI. Magnetic resonance imaging facilitates breast conservation for occult breast cancer. Ann Surg Oncol 2000; 7:411–415.

12

Carcinoma of Unknown Primary in a Single Site

Thierry Lesimple

Clinical Research Unit, Comprehensive Cancer Centre Eugène Marquis, Rennes, France

Carmen Balaña

Medical Oncology Service and Pathology Department, Institut Catalá D'Oncologia, Hospital Germans Trias i Pujol, Barcelona, Spain

INTRODUCTION

Carcinoma of unknown primary (CUP) in a single site accounts for about one-third of patients with CUP, and possibly represents a better prognosis than common forms. Differential diagnosis is particularly important, notably with a primary malignant tumor, and immunohistochemistry (IHC) can be especially helpful here. This entity justifies more extensive investigations (including positron emission tomography) than in disseminated forms, and such an approach may have an influence on the subsequent therapy for the patients. Local treatments (surgery, radiotherapy, etc.) are of particular importance when the metastasis is located in a single site, and chemotherapy (and/or hormone therapy for women in the event of positive hormonal receptors) may be considered even if its efficacy has not been fully evaluated in the literature.

Approximately one-third of the patients presenting with CUP have a unique metastatic site, corresponding by convention to a lymph-node involvement in only one area or a single visceral metastasis. The most frequent localizations are thus the liver, bones, lungs, and lymph nodes (1–3). In the study of Rades et al. of 42 patients with CUP in a single site, 34 patients presented with a lymph-node involvement and 8 showed a single visceral localization (bone 4, liver 2, pleura and central nervous system 1 in each) (4). Among these CUP occurring in a single site, some correspond to particular clinico-pathological entities (neuroendocrine or epidermoid histologies, peritoneal papillary serous carcinomatosis, or axillary lymph-node metastases in women) whose management is dealt with in Chapter 7. Moreover, as the frequency of CUP in the child is lower than 1% of diagnosed solid tumors, only CUP in the adult is discussed here (2).

The smaller the number of sites involved, the longer the survival of patients with CUP, especially if the lesion is potentially resectable (2): thus, the median overall survival is about 10 months when only one organ is involved, as against 6 months in the case of multiple involvement as in the population studied by Abbruzzese et al. (1). The survival is 20 months in the case of initially localized CUP, compared with 7 months in presentations that were disseminated at the outset, as found in the study of Hübner et al. (5). Free survival progression rates and overall survival rates are 83% and 87%, respectively, for the localized forms versus 33% and 47% for the disseminated forms. However, not all authors report the favorable prognosis of a single site of malignancy. In the study of van de Wouw et al., the beneficial influence of a unique site disappears in multivariate analysis at the expense of age, performance status, hepatic localization, and lactate dehydrogenase level (6).

DIFFERENTIAL DIAGNOSIS AND
PARACLINIC INVESTIGATIONS

One of the characteristic features of CUP at a single site is the importance of the differential diagnosis with a nontumoral pathology (in particular, of the infectious type), a benign tumor or, especially, a primary malignant tumor: pathological study and IHC can be of some help here, particularly in cases of undifferentiated histology. However, practically no marker is absolutely specific to a given histological type. In addition to electron microscopy and caryotype analysis (7), the role of molecular biology will certainly increase in importance. In this way, the gene expression profiling of metastases should allow a diagnosis of origin in 78% to more than 90% of cases, suggesting that tumors retain the markers of their tissue of origin throughout the process of metastatic evolution (8).

In this particular case, supplementary investigations should confirm the metastasis in a single localization and enable a more detailed search for a possible primary site. In addition to the examinations carried out systematically on CUP, as described elsewhere in this volume, it would appear reasonable to perform a spiral computed tomography (SCT) on the cerebral and thoraco-abdomino-pelvic regions, as well as a bone scan (9). Moreover, this should be combined with positron emission tomography using fluorine-18-fluorodeoxyglucose (PET-FDG), especially if aggressive surgery is considered with functional and/or aesthetic risks (10). Thus, in the study of Rades et al., PET-FDG identified the primary site in 43% of cases and pointed out a secondary dissemination in 38% of cases, in spite of the negative results of other common diagnostic procedures. Moreover, when the PET-FDG failed to find the primary tumor, it never appeared in later evolution. In total, for 29 patients out of 42 (69%), the result of PET-FDG had an influence on the subsequent therapeutic management. For 13 patients, the identification of the primary site led to a curative therapeutic approach, while, for 16 patients, dissemination of the disease was diagnosed only by PET-FDG and resulted in replacing the initial curative therapeutic strategy by palliative care (4).

To determine the best therapeutic strategy for a patient affected by a localized CUP, it is thus necessary to have the maximum amount of information on the occult primary tumor and the possible dissemination. Owing to a better prognosis than in the disseminated forms, local treatments (surgery, radiotherapy, etc.) can indeed take a particularly important place in this situation, where the patients can have a prolonged full remission. Chemotherapy should also be systematically discussed with patients in good general condition, even if its effectiveness is not evaluated in the literature. A few guidelines have been published on CUP with a unique site. Hormone therapy (and/or chemotherapy) of the type used in breast cancer may be discussed for women in the event of a positive result for hormonal receptors (progesterone and/or estrogen) within the tumor (11).

LOCALIZED LYMPH-NODE METASTASES OF A CUP

Some rare patients can present with a CUP involving a single lymph node (cervical, supraclavicular, axillary, inguinal, or mediastinal). The lymph-node localization is a favorable prognostic factor in CUP and a possible predictive factor of chemosensitivity, particularly for undifferentiated histologies (12). Prolonged survivals have been reported after excision of the lymph node with or without local radiation therapy (13,14). The diagnosis is made by fine needle aspiration cytology under echography, adenectomy, or lymph-node dissection, but a partial biopsy is contraindicated (15). In all cases, it may be interesting to perform a search for hormonal receptors (11).

The vast majority of cervical adenopathies are epidermoid and their management is addressed in Chapter 10. A cervical lymph-node metastasis of adenocarcinoma must be sought before a thyroid tumor by IHC [thyroglobulin, calcitonin (CT), thyroid transcription factor I (TTF-I)], cervical echography, serum assays for carcinoembryonic antigen and CT, or even exploratory cervicotomy. Cervical metastases of undifferentiated carcinomas should rule out the diagnosis of lymphoma or neuroendocrine tumors (12). Finally, undifferentiated carcinoma of the nasopharyngeal type should be evoked in the event of a characteristic context (9). Even if the survival rates for patients with these lymph-node malignancies is much lower than for epidermoid adenopathies, they should be treated by (selective) neck dissection and radiotherapy. However, there is no specific indication for systemic therapy (15).

Patients presenting with supraclavicular regional involvement have shorter survivals compared with those having other single-node localizations (1). In spite of the description of Troisier's ganglion, there is no difference in laterality or any indication of origin based on the side affected (9).

The management of localized axillary lymph node in women is dealt with elsewhere in this book. The involvement of isolated axillary lymph nodes in men does not require a specific assessment. The therapeutic approach suggested by the National Comprehensive Cancer Network comprises axillary lymph-node dissection followed by irradiation if two or more nodes are positive or in the event of extracapsular extension, possibly associated with chemotherapy (11).

The involvement of isolated inguinal nodes implies the removal of a melanoma, a lymphoma, or a urothelial carcinoma. It thus requires a careful exploration of the urogenital and anorectal areas (rectoscopy, colposcopy). As the axillary level, it justifies an inguinal lymph-node dissection with local irradiation if two or more nodes are affected or in the event of capsular rupture, and some patients have prolonged survivals (2).

The mediastinal lymph node (peribronchial, hilar, or mediastinal) metastases from a CUP have a poor prognosis. When they are isolated, the occult primary tumor is commonly pulmonary and seldom located below the diaphragm (16). Such a localization requires mediastinoscopy aimed at diagnosis, and histological examination should rule out a small-cell lung cancer. However, the latter can be presented only in the form of mediastinal adenopathies that are accessible to a treatment with a curative objective. An undifferentiated malignant tumor in a young man should also allow the ruling out of an extragonadic germ cell tumor (9). The diagnostic mediastinoscopy should be followed by chemotherapy and then, if excision of the nodes is technically possible, by mediastinal lymph-node dissection. This procedure may be associated with resection of the adjacent pulmonary parenchyma if necessary. The alternative is to carry out a thoracotomy at the outset with a diagnostic and therapeutic purpose, if the dissection appears feasible, followed by chemotherapy. In all cases, the dissection must be extended to all the lymph-node chains concerned on the same side of the mediastinum. A complementary mediastinal irradiation is indicated, at least in the event of incomplete lymph-node dissection (17). Prolonged survivals have thus been described when resection was possible.

LIVER METASTASIS FROM A CUP IN A SINGLE SITE

Although exclusively liver malignancies account for approximately 25% of liver metastases of CUP, they seldom occur in a single site (18). The essential procedure is a liver biopsy (19) and the predominant histology is adeno-carcinoma (20,21).

The differential diagnosis between a poorly differentiated hepato-cellular carcinoma and a cholangiocellular carcinoma is relatively easy with IHC and alpha-fetoprotein assays, just as with the diagnosis of metastases from colo-rectal carcinoma, even if there are paradoxical IHC profiles (3). On the other hand, it is practically impossible to distinguish between a cholangiocellular carcinoma and a metastase from a gastric or a pancreatic adenocarcinoma, even by means of IHC (9). Moreover, it is particularly important to identify the hepatic metastatic localization of a neuroendocrine carcinoma, since its prognosis may be better (19). The use of cytokeratins (CK) 7 and 20 is helpful in the case of a CK20+ profile, but the majority of CUP are CK20− and the primary site cannot be accurately predicted (20). It is legitimate to propose a coloscopy in the case of a CK20+/CK7− profile to research a primary colo-rectal adenocarcinoma. This is because these lesions have a prevalent colo-rectal origin and are by defini-tion amenable to a loco-regional treatment (surgical resection, intra-arterial chemotherapy, or chemoembolization) (18). Whether an endoscopic cholan-giopancreatography and/or an endoscopic ultrasound should be carried out in the case of a CK20+/CK7+ profile to rule out a biliary or pancreatic adenocarcinoma (21) is more debatable because the identification of such primary tumors may not dramatically change therapeutic management.

While a few patients present with an isolated single hepatic localiza-tion, survival seems barely higher than for patients with multiple hepatic metastases or with associated extrahepatic localizations (median of survival of about four months), thus perhaps not justifying any difference in thera-peutic approach from other CUP (18,19). A liver localization is indeed particularly pejorative in CUP (13).

Hepatic resection has a well-established place in treating hepatic metastases of colo-rectal cancer or neuroendocrine tumors, just as with radiofrequency ablation, and both techniques have a low morbidity and mortality. The extrapolation to CUP with resectable hepatic metastases remains a matter of debate and a few cases are reported in the literature (22). In the study of Berney et al., the local recurrences are frequent and mainly remain limited to the liver (23). Other local treatments can be discussed, including chemoembolization, hepatic artery infusion, etc. Hepatic localiza-tions are also less sensitive to systemic treatments (24), while chemotherapy would appear especially useful for differentiated metastases of adenocarci-nomas (25). Some authors would thus favor a chemotherapy adapted to colo-rectal, pulmonary, or pancreatic tumors (11,21).

ISOLATED BONE METASTASIS

Single bone metastases account for up to 22% of patients with metastatic bony lesions. In the absence of extraskeletal localizations, this justifies investigations in more detail when there are multiple bone metastases. Ten to fifty percent of the osseous metastatic patients present with tumors of unknown primary site, including a large majority of differentiated or undifferentiated carcinomas (26,27).

The sclerotic character of the lesion should orient diagnosis toward a prostate origin, justifying recourse to a prostate biopsy under ultrasound guidance. However, as bone metastases from prostate cancer may not always be radiologically osteoblastic, it seems practically logical to recommend a rectal digital examination and a serum prostate specific antigen (PSA) in all men with bone metastases from a CUP. The localization of the lesion and its radiological aspect may also evoke a particular origin or a primary bone tumor. In the case of single localization, serum and urine protein electrophoresis is useful in ruling out a plasmocytoma (28). The other serum markers are of more debatable interest (2). Neither bone scans, SCT or magnetic resonance imaging (MRI), of the lesion can provide assistance for identifying the primary (26).

Biopsy under the guidance of X ray or SCT, or better open surgical biopsy, can confirm the malignity. The alternative is to perform an initial fine-needle aspiration biopsy, which allowed a diagnosis in 93% of cases in the study of Wedin et al. These authors continued their investigations as a function of the cytological results (29). The localization in a single site also justifies the carrying out of an osteomedullary biopsy to rule out a microscopic dissemination. Above all, the occurrence of metastases in a single site imposes a surgical biopsy because a curative treatment is possible (26). The placement of the biopsy incision is critical because, if the final diagnosis were a primary bone tumor, this would then generally require a subsequent resection and reconstruction. A biopsy carried out incorrectly on a patient with a primary bone tumor can lead to an amputation, whereas the patient would have been a candidate for limb salvage surgery. The same problem arises in the case of an inaugural pathological fracture requiring a needle biopsy or a surgical biopsy to rule out the diagnosis of a primary bone tumor before carrying out osteosynthesis (28). IHC studies can indicate tumors with common skeletal metastatic site that are accessible to an effective treatment (PSA, alpha-fetoprotein, CT, and thyroglobulin) and can be used to rule out a primary bone tumor: osteosarcoma, lymphoma, Ewing's sarcoma before 40 years and, more rarely, malignant fibrous histiocytoma of bone and chondrosarcoma, as well as primary lymphoma of bone and plasmocytoma in older patients. These the last two diagnoses seldom require a surgical treatment (1,28,29).

In cases of extravertebral involvement in a patient in good general condition, prophylactic surgery resection is indicated, the alternative being an external radiotherapy (11). It is difficult to know if complementary irradiation is necessary after a surgical resection, except if this latter is incomplete or limiting. Otherwise, metabolic radiotherapy (Strontium-89, Samarium-153) has no place in the treatment of a single lesion. Bone metastases are also classically rather insensitive to chemotherapy (24), although this assumption might be related to the fact that response to chemotherapy is difficult to assess radiologically in bone lesions. The use of diphosphonates can be considered as a anti-osteoclastic by analogy with other cancers, even though there are very few data in the literature (13). These drugs allow an improvement of the quality of life, leading to a reduction in the number of bone incidents and the number of radiotherapy sequences, while decreasing the risk of hypercalcemia (27). Here again, the single-site character of the lesion makes such a treatment debatable.

In addition to standard radiographies of the rachis and a bone scan, a vertebral metastasis with unknown primary site justifies an SCT and an MRI of the involved vertebra to specify the extent of osseous and spinal canal involvement (30). The assessment would also include an osteomedullary biopsy and a complete vertebral MRI, from C0 to S5, to identify any other vertebrae involved.

With vertebral involvement in a single site, a surgical excision must be carried out if possible, preceded by a spinal arteriography in the event of lower thoracic or upper lumbar involvement with a view sufficient for embolizing the neoplastic vessels. A higher cervical or thoracic lesion contraindicates an embolization by systemic route and requires a percutaneous embolization (30). An alternative to surgery is offered by cementoplasty. In all cases, antalgic radiotherapy has a central role to play.

On the whole, while patients with bone-located CUP have a short survival of the order of five months (27), this can be much longer in cases of isolated bone metastasis from a renal or thyroid primary occult site, which can justify an extensive resection and reconstructive surgery (28–30).

SOLITARY PULMONARY NODULE FROM A CUP

Fifty to sixty percent of single pulmonary nodules are benign (infectious granulomas), this percentage varying with the age of the patient, the size and localization of the lesion, and smoking history. The most advantageous strategy for selecting indications for more invasive explorations involves associating a thoracic SCT with PET-FDG, even if the latter technique can yield false negatives (tumors smaller than 6–8 mm) or false positives (tuberculosis, histoplasmosis, and abscess). The diagnosis of malignity can be confirmed by transthoracic needle aspiration biopsy, fibre-optic bronchoscopy, video-assisted thoracoscopy, thoracotomy, or video-assisted thoracoscopic surgery (31). Fine-needle aspiration biopsy and thoracoscopy are the most commonly employed techniques.

The principal differential diagnosis is the primary lung cancer, which is impossible to obtain on a standard radiography (2) and not always straight-forward, even with an IHC study (9): only 9% to 15% of lung cancers express CK20, which is useful in differentiating primary tumors from pulmonary metastases of adenocarcinomas. On the other hand, 85% of primary lung cancers express CK7, so the use of TTF-I and surfactant apoprotein allows us to differentiate them from other CK7$^+$ tumors, but not from malignant mesotheliomas: TTF-I has a specificity of 95% to 100% and a sensitivity of 65% for lung primary tumors and cadherin E has a sensitivity of 100% (8).

Thus, in the case of an adenocarcinoma or undifferentiated pulmonary carcinoma that is isolated or without any other orientation, it is a general rule to regard it as a primary pulmonary carcinoma and treat it as such (1).

LOCALIZED PLEURAL EFFUSION OF A CUP

Five to fifteen percent of metastatic pleural effusions are of unknown primary site, which, for some authors, justifies the individualization of a specific entity termed "primary intrathoracic malignant effusion" (32). Some of these tumors probably also originate from small subpleural carcinomas ("pseudomesothelio-matous carcinoma of the lung") corresponding to peripheral adenocarcinomas of the lung with extensive pleural growth and little peripheral parenchymal involvement (33). The large majority of patients presenting with metastatic pleural effusions of unknown primary site do not have a smoking history. Pathology is generally indicative of an adenocarcinoma, with two-thirds of cases showing pleura as the single site of metastasis. The principal differential diagnosis is pleural mesothelioma. Survival is 10 months in this isolated group as against 7 months in cases of associated extrapleural localization (34).

Pleural fluid cytology can be sufficient to confirm the malignity and rule out a diagnosis of mesothelioma in 58% of cases. The sensitivity of closed pleural biopsies is lower (33). Medical thoracoscopy (under local anesthesia and analgesia) and surgical thoracoscopy (under general anesthe-sia with selective intubation) can offer a wide range of advantages here, both in diagnosis (extensive biopsies under direct observation) as well as in symp-tomatic therapy (talc pleurodesis) with a sensitivity of 95% (9). In difficult diagnoses, IHC studies (TTF-I, calretinin) can differentiate an adenocarci-noma from a mesothelioma. After evacuation, it is justified to practice an SCT of the thorax, but if the SCT does not show an anomaly, the fibre-optic bronchoscopy is always negative and will thus be ineffective (32).

Local treatment by drainage, shunt, or sclerosing therapy only has a pal-liative effect in the short term, with a high risk of reconstitution of the effusion (32). Major surgery such as parietal pleurectomy, decortication, or pleurop-neumonectomy does not prove more efficacious in palliative terms. The cura-tive benefit of such operations is not demonstrated even in cases of primary intrathoracic malignant effusion. Perioperative mortality is high and this type of surgery should only be discussed among highly selected patients. When the disease is localized in the pleural cavity, intrapleural chemotherapy may treat the underlying neoplasm in addition to controlling the effusion. Pseudo-mesotheliomatous carcinomas of the lung are also among the most ideal targets for this type of local treatment. Systemic chemotherapy seems to have a positive effect on the symptoms and maybe on overall survival (34). Finally, as always, the quality of life is of crucial importance for these patients, in particular the control of dyspnea and pain (33).

SINGLE CEREBRAL METASTASIS OF A CUP

Up to 15% of cerebral metastases are of unknown primary site. The median of survival is 9 to 14 months after surgery and radiotherapy in the majority of the studies, with overall survival rates of 30% to 57% at one year and 19% to 25% at two years (35–37). From one-third to one-half of the patients have a single lesion, with adenocarcinoma being the most frequent histology (38,39). The single localization of the lesion can only be confirmed by MRI, particularly in the case of lesions in the posterior fossa or multiple punctate metastases. The localization thus determined is frontal in 25% of cases, parietal in 25%, and cerebellar in 25%, this last localization appearing to be more frequent in the population of CUP (40). Certain characteristics on the SCT or MRI are indicative of a metastasis, but none of them is pathognomonic: peripheral location, spherical shape, ring enhancement, and prominent peritumoral edema. In the event of a single localization proved by MRI, a craniotomy must be carried out to perform a complete resection when this is possible. If not, a biopsy is essential in order to rule out a benign pathology (abscess, infection, or hemorrhage) or a primary cerebral tumor (glioma, lymphoma) (41). In the case of an undifferentiated malignant tumor, IHC (glial fibrillary acidic protein, neurofilaments, etc.) can be very useful to exclude the possibility of a primary cerebral tumor (9). Otherwise, examination of the cerebrospinal fluid becomes essential in the event of any signs evoking carcinomatous meningitis (42).

The survival rates of patients with cerebral metastases of unknown primary in a single site is higher than that for patients having multiple localizations: in the study of Salvati et al., it is 43% at one year and 19% at two years (median = 32 months) (40), with some long-term survivors beyond five years (38,41). However, the resectability is a more important prognostic factor than the single localization of the lesion (39), and another prognostic factor is the Karnofsky preoperative index (42).

Three randomized studies have shown that patients with a single lesion and treated by complete resection before whole-brain radiotherapy (WBRT) have less local recurrences, better survival, and better quality of life than in cases with WBRT alone, without high mortality related to the surgery (35,36,43). Thus, surgery should be considered in any patient with a single brain metastasis in an accessible location, when the size is large, the mass effect is significant and/or an obstructive hydrocephalus is present. Complete surgical resection allows an immediate relief of symptoms of intracranial hypertension and seizures, a reduction of focal neurological deficits, and a rapid steroid taper in the majority of patients. In the event of an exclusive local recurrence in a patient in good performance status, a reoperation may also allow a neurological improvement and a prolongation of survival. In the same way, when the number of metastases is limited (generally up to three), and the lesions are accessible, with a young patient in good general and neurological condition, complete surgical resection yields similar results to those for single lesions (42). Finally, the resection of a symptomatic lesion and the radiation treatment of the other ones is of clinical value as well (37).

An alternative is stereotaxic radiosurgery (SRS), because only a minority of single cerebral metastases are accessible to surgery (35). Single cerebral metastases are indeed ideal targets for SRS. They are generally small, spherical, minimally invasive, and show radiographically distinct margins. SRS allows a rapid decrease of symptoms, local control rates of 80% to 90% of cases, and a median survival ranging from 7 to 12 months. Favorable factors for long-term control include a diameter of less than 3 cm, homogeneous baseline enhancement, and a good initial radiographic response to SRS. Moreover, metastases classically radioresistant to fractionated radiotherapy seem to respond to SRS as well as the tumors known to be radiosensitive. Thus, the SRS allows an effective treatment of patients presenting with comorbidities or with an inaccessible lesion. In the absence of extracerebral disease, SRS on its own or associated with WBRT seems to be better than conventional irradiation in terms of local control, survival, and quality of life. The results are indeed comparable with those reported for surgery associated with WBRT (42). Finally, the early or late complications are relatively moderate after treatment of a cerebral metastasis by SRS.

While adjuvant WBRT after surgery improves local control and decreases the risk of new cerebral metastases at remote sites, its utility remains a matter of debate. Indeed, it is responsible for early adverse effects (fatigue, alopecia, and Eustachian tube dysfunction) and late neurotoxicity in 5% of cases (37,40). The total dose and the fractions are thus important factors to be taken into account: the patients with an a priori favorable prognosis should be treated with conventional fractions from 1.8 to 2 Gy to a total dose of 40 to 50 Gy. However, the current tendency is not to perform adjuvant WBRT after surgery, especially if the lesion is radioresistant, but rather to reserve the WBRT or SRS for the recurrence. Certain treatment centres simply carry out a focal irradiation after surgical resection (42). In all cases, WBRT should not be used on it own in this indication except if there is a contraindication with the surgery and the SRS.

The status of chemotherapy in this context is more debatable, because these localizations are only weakly chemosensitive apart from some particular histological forms (42).

On the whole, an aggressive approach associating surgical resection or SRS with or without WBRT is justified for patients with an isolated single cerebral metastasis of unknown primary site, and very prolonged survivals are possible (38,41). After local treatment by surgery or SRS, overall survival does not seem affected if the WBRT is reserved for the later recurrence (42).

METASTASIS OF CUTANEOUS OR SOFT TISSUES FROM A CUP

These localizations theoretically have a better prognosis (13). The differential diagnosis of a single cutaneous metastatic localization corresponds to melanoma, particularly when it is achromic. In the event of cutaneous metastasis of an undifferentiated carcinoma, the ruling out of a Merkel cell carcinoma is facilitated by an IHC study (chromogranin A, CK20, neurofilaments, etc.) (9).

The presentation of a solitary metastasis in soft tissues (subcutaneous tissue and skeletal muscle) is a rare occurrence, accounting for approximately 2.5% of the tumors of soft tissues, among which 0.8% are of unknown primary site. The diagnosis should exclude the possibility of a benign lesion (hematoma, infection), a sarcoma, or a melanoma (44). MRI is the preferred technique for characterizing these lesions, but it is often difficult to rule out a primary sarcoma of the soft tissues. Because of this, a biopsy is required to take this diagnosis into account.

CONCLUSION

A small group of patients presenting with a CUP have a single metastatic localization that remains isolated, even if an exhaustive assessment is performed (and even if this assessment includes a PET-FDG). According to the site concerned, a radical local treatment by surgical resection and/or irradiation should be discussed. The majority of the patients in fact show some benefit in palliative terms, and some have a prolonged free interval before the appearance of other metastatic sites. On the other hand, there is no data available making it possible to recommend or disfavor the use of systemic chemotherapy.

REFERENCES

1. Abbruzzese JL, Abbruzzese MC, Hess KR, Raber MN, Lenzi R, Frost P. Unknown primary carcinoma: natural history and prognostic factors in 657 consecutive patients. J Clin Oncol 1994; 12:1272–1280.
2. Pavlidis N, Briasoulis E, Hainsworth J, Greco FA. Diagnostic and therapeutic management of cancer of an unknown primary. Eur J Cancer 2003; 39: 1990–2005.

3. Belleannée G. Tumeurs sans primitif connu: place de l'immunohistochimie. Oncologie 2004; 6:252–255.
4. Rades D, Kuhnel G, Wildfang I, Borner AR, Schmoll HJ, Knapp W. Localised disease in cancer of unknown primary (CUP): the value of positron emission tomography (PET) for individual therapeutic management. Ann Oncol 2001; 12:1605–1609.
5. Hübner G, Wildfang I, Schmoll HJ. CUP. In: Schmoll HJ, ed. Kompendium Internistische Onkologie Band 2. Berlin/Heidelberg/New York: Springer-Verlag, 1999:2137–2182.
6. van de Wouw AJ, Jansen RLH, Griffioen AW, Hillen HFP. Clinical and immunohistochemical analysis of patients with unknown primary tumour. A search for prognostic factors in UPT. Anticancer Res 2004; 24:297–302.
7. Pénel N. Prise en charge diagnostique des métastases inaugurales. Presse Med 2003; 32:990–996.
8. Varadhachary GR, Abbruzzese JL, Lenzi R. Diagnostic strategies for unknown primary cancer. Cancer 2004; 100:1776–1785.
9. Lesimple T, Voigt JJ, Bataillard A, et al. Recommandations pour la pratique clinique: Standards, Options et Recommandations 2002 pour le diagnostic des carcinomes de site primitif inconnu. Bull Cancer 2003; 90:1071–1096.
10. Lassen U, Daugaard G, Eigtved A, Damgaard K, Friberg L. 18F-FDG whole body positron emission tomography (PET) in patients with unknown primary tumours (UPT). Eur J Cancer 1999; 35:1076–1082.
11. Anonymous. NCCN practice guidelines for occult primary tumours. National Comprehensive Cancer Network. Oncology 1998; 12:226–309.
12. Pénel N. Pronostic et possibilités thérapeutiques des métastases inaugurales. Presse Med 2003; 32:997–1004.
13. Bugat R, Bataillard A, Lesimple T, et al. Summary of the standards, options and recommendations for the management of patients with carcinoma of unknown primary site. Br J Cancer 2003; 89(suppl 1):S59–S66.
14. Hainsworth JD, Greco FA. Treatment of patients with cancer of an unknown primary site. N Engl J Med 1993; 329:257–263.
15. Zuur CL, van Velthuysen MLF, Schornagel JH, Hilgers FJM, Balm AJM. Diagnosis and treatment of isolated neck metastases of adenocarcinomas. Eur J Surg Oncol 2002; 28:147–152.
16. Riquet M, Badoual C, le Pimpec Barthes F, Dujon A, Danel C. Metastatic thoracic lymph node carcinoma with unknown primary site. Ann Thorac Surg 2003; 75:244–249.
17. Faure E, Riquet M, Lombe-Weta PM, Hübsch JP, Carnot F. Adénopathies tumorales du médiastin sans cancer primitif. Rev Mal Respir 2000; 17:1095–1099.
18. Mousseau M, Schaerer R, Lutz JM, Ménégoz F, Faure H, Swiercz P. Métastases hépatiques de site primitif inconnu. Bull Cancer 1991; 78:725–736.
19. Hogan BA, Thornton FJ, Brannigan M, et al. Hepatic metastases from an unknown primary neoplasm (UPN): survival, prognostic indicators and value of extensive investigations. Clin Radiol 2002; 57:1073–1077.
20. Tot T, Samii S. The clinical relevance of cytokeratin phenotyping in needle biopsy of liver metastasis. APMIS 2003; 111:1075–1082.

21. Hawksworth J, Geisinger K, Zagoria R, et al. Surgical and ablative treatment for metastatic adenocarcinoma to the liver from unknown primary tumor. Am Surg 2004; 70:512–517.

22. Schwartz SI. Hepatic resection for noncolorectal nonneuroendocrine metastases. World J Surg 1995; 19:72–75.

23. Berney T, Mentha G, Roth AD, Morel P. Results of surgical resection of liver metastases from non-colorectal primaries. Br J Surg 1998; 85:1423–1427.

24. Briasoulis E, Kalofonos H, Bafaloukos D, et al. Carboplatin plus paclitaxel in unknown primary carcinoma: a phase II Hellenic Cooperative Oncology Group Study. J Clin Oncol 2000; 18:3101–3107.

25. Ayoub JP, Hess KR, Abbruzzese MC, Lenzi R, Raber MN, Abbruzzese JL. Unknown primary tumors metastatic to liver. J Clin Oncol 1998; 16:2105–2112.

26. Alcalay M, Azais I, Brigeon B, et al. Strategy for identifying primary malignancies with inaugural bone metastases. Rev Rhum Engl Ed 1995; 62:632–642.

27. Conroy T, Platini C, Troufléau P, et al. Présentation clinique et facteurs pronostiques au diagnostic de métastases osseuses. A propos d'une série de 578 observations. Bull Cancer 1993; 80(suppl 10):16–22.

28. Rougraff BT. Evaluation of the patient with carcinoma of unknown origin metastatic to bone. Clin Orthop 2003; 415(suppl):S105–S109.

29. Wedin R, Bauer HCF, Skoog L, Söderlund V, Tani E. Cytological diagnosis of skeletal lesions. Fine-needle aspiration biopsy in 110 tumours. J Bone Joint Surg Br 2000; 82:673–678.

30. Enkaoua EA, Doursounian L, Chatellier G, Mabesoone F, Aimard T, Saillant G. Vertebral metastases: a critical appreciation of the preoperative prognostic Tokuhashi score in a series of 71 cases. Spine 1997; 22:2293–2298.

31. Gambhir SS, Shepherd JE, Shah BD, et al. Analytical decision model for the cost-effective management of solitary pulmonary nodules. J Clin Oncol 1998; 16:2113–2125.

32. Bonnefoi H, Smith IE. How should cancer presenting as a malignant pleural effusion be managed? Br J Cancer 1996; 74:832–835.

33. Antony VB, Loddenkemper R, Astoul P, et al. Management of malignant pleural effusions. Eur Respir J 2001; 18:402–419.

34. Ang P, Tan EH, Leong SS, et al. Primary intrathoracic malignant effusion: a descriptive study. Chest 2001; 120:50–54.

35. Patchell RA, Tibbs PA, Walsh JW, et al. A randomized trial of surgery in the treatment of single metastases to the brain. N Engl J Med 1990; 322:494–500.

36. Vecht CJ, Haaxma-Reiche H, Noordijk EM, et al. Treatment of single brain metastasis: radiotherapy alone or combined with neurosurgery? Ann Neurol 1993; 33:583–590.

37. Rudà R, Borgognone M, Benech F, Vasario E, Soffietti R. Brain metastases from unknown primary tumour: a prospective study. J Neurol 2001; 248:394–398.

38. Nguyen LN, Maor MH, Oswald MJ. Brain metastases as the only manifestation of an undetected primary tumor. Cancer 1998; 83:2181–2184.

39. Bartelt S, Lutterbach J. Brain metastases in patients with cancer of unknown primary. J Neurooncol 2003; 64:249–253.

40. Salvati M, Cervoni L, Raco A. Single brain metastases from unknown primary malignancies in CT-era. J Neurooncol 1995; 23:75–80.

41. Khansur T, Routh A, Hickman B. Brain metastases from unknown primary site. J Miss State Med Assoc 1997; 38:238–242.
42. Soffietti R, Rudà R, Mutani R. Management of brain metastases. J Neurol 2002; 249:1357–1369.
43. Mintz AH, Kestle J, Rathbone MP, et al. A randomized trial to assess the efficacy of surgery in addition to radiotherapy in patients with a single cerebral metastasis. Cancer 1996; 78:1470–1476.
44. Glockner JF, White LM, Sundaram M, McDonald DJ. Unsuspected metastases presenting as solitary soft tissue lesions: a fourteen-year review. Skeletal Radiol 2000; 29:270–274.

13

Emerging Local Treatments in Carcinomas of an Unknown Primary Site: Radiofrequency, Palliative Bone Surgery, and Radiotherapy

D. Pasquier and E. Lartigau
Department of Radiation Oncology, Centre O. Lambret,
University Lille II, Lille, France

F. Bonodeau
Department of Radiology, Centre O. Lambret, Lille, France

G. Missenard
Department of Surgery, Clinique Arago, Paris, France

C. Court
Department of Orthopaedic Surgery, Kremlin Bicêtre Hospital,
Paris Sud University, Paris, Leclerc, France

B. Meunier
Department of Oncological Surgery, Pontchaillou Hospital , Rennes, France

INTRODUCTION

Carcinomas of an unknown primary (CUP) site represent about 3% to 5% of all cancer types (1–4). New local treatments have occurred in metastatic disease but there are a few specific CUP-related data. Several techniques will be developed in a broader framework. In this chapter, we will discuss radiofrequency, which is now part of the local treatment of hepatic metastases, whereas extracerebral stereotactic radiotherapy should be initiated soon. Concerning bone metastases, a unique radiotherapy session allows the same antalgic effect and, as durable as hypofractioned patterns. Surgery, particularly in the preventive indications, plays an important role in the treatment of these secondary bone lesions. In the future, trials specific to CUP should be considered in order to better specify the indications and the efficiency of these treatments.

Squamous cell carcinoma of an unknown primary located in the head and neck and the operable lesions after chemotherapy treatments are specific entities and will not be discussed in this chapter.

RADIOFREQUENCY

If the gold standard of hepatic metastases local treatment is still the surgical ablation, new methods of tumor destruction could improve the treatment of nonoperable tumors, either because of a bilobar location or because of an anesthetic contraindication.

In addition to the chemical destruction by intratumoral injection, lesions can be destroyed by heat, essentially laser thermal rise, radiofrequence, or freezing, i.e., cryonics. These last two methods are the most widespread and benefit from ambulatory implementation; the technique based on the radiofrequency waves is the mostly used.

The destruction principle lies on the ionic disturbances of the tissue crossed by a sinusoidal current having a 400 to 500 Hz frequency (5). Because of particles friction, the tissue warms up to 60°C resulting in a coagulation necrosis. The spreading lesion starting from the electrode leads to a sphere, the size of which is determined by the active electrode size, the intensity, and the duration of the current passage.

Two types of electrodes are used: either a simple electrode with a single or stand-used end, or a retractable electrode spreading as an umbrella with a variable number of ribs. The cooling system for the electrode end avoids the carbonization phenomenon noticed at a temperature of 80°C and by blocking the current transmission, it ends in the nondestruction of the lesion.

This technique is often performed with a general anesthesia and antibiotic prophylaxis. The lesion is located by ultrasonography, either by transcutaneous method or during surgery. The treatment is monitored by ultrasonography, computed tomography (CT), or magnetic resonance imaging (MRI). In addition, this technique benefits from vascular clamping or cooling the bile ducts for lesions located close to sensitive areas.

The contraindications are more than four hepatic lesions, lesion larger than 5 cm in diameter, presence of a bilious-digestive anastomosis, contact to the bladder, colon, or stomach when it is about a percutaneous duct, and coagulation disturbances. The morbidity varies from 3% to 15%; in a recent survey Curley et al. reports 7% immediate complications and 2.4% late complications (6). A postablation syndrome associating pain, fever, and nauseas can be noticed. Equally intrahepatic or subcapsular hematoma related to the electrode crossing, infarction by vascular thromboses or cholecystitis can be noticed. Later, intrahepatic abscesses and bile ducts stenosis may occur. Rhim et al. report 10% to 20% of recurrences mainly because of the nonobservance of security margin around lesions (7).

Cryotherapy is based on the destruction of tumor cells by fast freezing at −20°C. This method relies on the implementation of one or several liquid nitrogen operating cryosurgical probes. Using several probes enables the destruction of large lesions up to 8 cm. The overall destructed volume should not exceed 200 cm^2 in order to avoid shocks that are the main cause of postoperative mortality, about 1.5%. The recurrence rates vary from 33% for Siefert et al. to 9% for Ruers et al. (8,9). Finally, Goering et al. report a recurrence rate comparable to that of the surgical resection for noncolorectal metastases (10). This technique is more difficult than radiofrequency, limiting its development.

These data are chiefly based on the treatment of metastases from gastrointestinal tract cancers. A few data on the CUP are available. A recent retrospective survey of Hawksworth et al. reports the evolution of 7 patients treated by radiofrequency or surgery from hepatic lesions of an adenocarcinoma of unknown primary, in a series of 157 patients. Out of nine lesions, six were treated by radiofrequency, one patient had extrahepatic lesions before the treatment. The median recurrence-free survival was 6.5 months (11).

The radiofrequency may be part of the local treatment for hepatic metastases; the criteria for patients' selection have to be similar to the surgical ones. The radiofrequency indications arise from the surgical contraindications as the procedure seems less invasive with lower morbidity rate due to smaller resections, protecting the hepatic function or making the operation easier.

PALLIATIVE BONE SURGERY

More than half of the patients affected by a CUP have bone metastases (12). Treating the bone metastases has to be multidisciplinary; local treatments such as radiotherapy and surgery may be added to the systemic treatment. The orthopedic surgery has lately gained an important role in the treatment of bone metastases of limbs and spine, regardless of their origin. Today the improvements in the arthroplasty and osteosynthesis allow a fast and efficient treatment. Pain, pathological fractures, and neurological disturbances must be avoided for patient's quality of life. One of the major difficulties is to indicate a preventive intervention (13,14).

The main goal of this type of surgery is to remove tumor and to consolidate the bone. The surgical strategy should avoid discomfort and the subsequent decubitus-related postoperative complications in order to enable a rapid social reintegration.

Technically, a direct approach of the lesion would be preferable in order to remove tumor and to fix the material in healthy bone. Histological sampling has to be systematic. Surgery may be hemorrhagic and can be preceded by embolization. The osteosynthesis or the arthroplasty has to protect the entire corresponding bone segment in order to avoid the discovery of another weak area. It implies an adequate preoperative check-up with X rays of the entire bone segment for limbs and with MRI of the entire vertebral axis for the rachis. For limbs and waist the substance loss will be filled with acrylic cement that may be replaced by bone grafts for spine surgery.

There are three types of therapeutic indications: the known metastatic patients with a large or hyperalgetic lesion, a prefracture mechanical weakening, and/or by a neurological threat. These three situations are often combined particularly at the spine level. In this case, a preventive treatment is essential. Patients were examined for either a pathological fracture, in spite of an adequate medical treatment, or a revealing fracture. In this particular case, it is essential to be histologically certain before planning an adapted strategy. Finally, the patients with a single bone metastasis may benefit from oncologic surgery, in very specific situations. Obviously, one has to be certain that this lesion is isolated by a complete extension check-up. The surgical strategy has to be considered depending on locations.

Limbs and Waist

One should distinguish between the preventive and curative fracture treatment. Before the fracture, the anatomic changes are minimum, the bone or articular stabilization will be easy to perform and solid, resulting in limited sequels with a better antalgic and functional result. The diagnosis of a prefracture state is clinical with a recrudescence of pain during rest, becoming resistant to major antalgic treatment. CT and MRI are useful to view a 3-D extension. Classically, there is a pathological fracture risk when the lesions concern more than a third of the long bone diameter. In this case, the anatomic–clinical confrontation should result in a preventive surgical indication. After any fracture, the surgical indication is critical as spontaneous consolidation rate is low. The emergency situation gives a higher morbidity ratio (15–18).

The unique lesion should be assessed individually as oncologic surgery may be a good recourse. Oncologic surgery is obviously more aggressive than palliative surgery but modern reconstruction procedures, especially massive prosthesis implant operations, allow a functional result and a fast and satisfactory rehabilitation.

Spine

At this level the clinical presentation will be different but preventive surgery remains essential. The pathological fracture is more difficult to foresee and it is not a formal contraindication to the medical treatment. It will be difficult to appreciate the neurological risk and the disease extension on the entire rachis. MRI is essential to get the right information on these lesions. It should include a sagittal sequence showing the entire axis in order to plan surgery. Moreover, the surgical indications may be classified in two types: preventive and curative.

Preventive Treatment

1. Unstable lesion for which stabilization is indicated in order to make the adjuvant treatments easier. In this case, a posterior stabilization remains simple and efficient due to the new titanium-made instruments allowing an easy monitoring with MRI (Fig. 1) (19).
2. Large lesion, resisting to medical treatment and triggering a mechanical and neurological risk: corporeal lesions needing an anterior approach with corporectomy that is a simple act at the cervical rachis level but more difficult in the dorsal–lumbar region. However, the contribution of less invasive techniques such as thoracoscopy at the dorsal level allows enlarging these indications without increasing the morbidity ratio.
3. Discovery of a threatening epidural lesion may need a preventive decompression before the appearance of neurological disturbances. In these cases, it is most often laminectomy, which carries the risk of aggravating the vertebral instability needing a vertebral stabilization (20).

Treatment of Complications

1. Neurological disturbances seriously endanger the success rate of the intervention, and the existence of a completely installed paraplegia at the dorsal level may be a surgical contraindication as there are very few chances for recuperation.
2. Total vertebrectomy is an exceptional indication concerning either isolated lesions or slowly progressive forms. The progress of imaging and the rachidian stabilization give a good success rate for these interventions.

Therefore, a multidisciplinary approach should ensure the best therapeutic sequence. One has to emphasize the importance of a preventive strategy, giving significantly better results. In these cases, the surgery of bone metastases is very efficient and significantly improves quality of life.

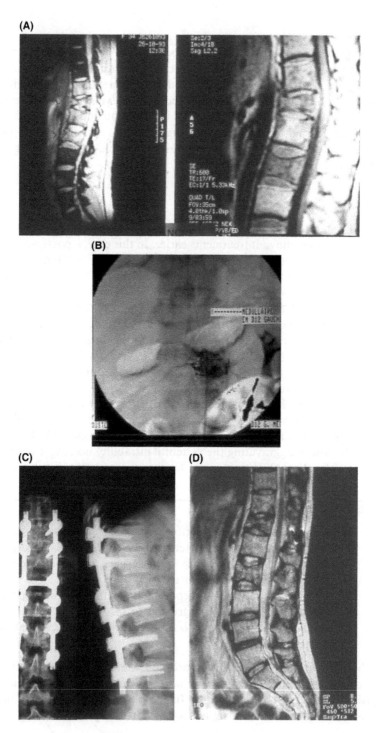

Figure 1 (*Caption on facing page.*)

RADIOTHERAPY

Pain, a moderate fracture risk and a medullar compression, are the most common indications of radiotherapy for bone metastases. The goals of radiotherapy are to improve the symptoms, to restore the function, and to prevent the effects of tumor progress in the treated area with moderate side effects. The methods of this palliative radiotherapy should observe rules, such as performing a simulation of the treatment enabling the definition of the treated areas with the help of the clinical examination and radiological data (bone scan, standard X rays, and CT). Similar to surgery, the nuclear magnetic resonance is the reference examination for rachis exploration.

In most of the cases, the antalgic radiotherapy is performed according to a hypofractioned regime (dose per fraction above 2 Gy) in order to shorten the treatment duration. The efficacy of the antalgic radiotherapy is linked to an anti-tumor effect, but also to an anti-inflammatory effect, with the destruction of the macrophagic cells at the origin of the production of cytokines pain mediation like the prostaglandin E_2 (21). The patterns used in North America and Europe are 10 sessions of 3 Gy or 5 to 6 sessions of 4 Gy (22,23), giving objective and complete response of about 70% and 30% (24,25). Many trials dealt with the efficiency of a unique session. There are few data on the metastases of unknown primary. Steenland et al., in a randomized trial including more than 1100 patients, compare on the efficiency of a 8 Gy session with 6 × 4 Gy-sessions. Approximately 90% of patients were affected by breast, prostate, or lung cancer. The affected bone locations were the pelvis, the rachis, and the lower limbs respectively. The patients having a medullar compression or a pathological fracture were excluded. The response to radiotherapy was defined as a decrease higher or equal to two of the analogical visual score; the patients were considered in complete response if they did not have any pain regardless of the antalgic consumption. The partial and complete response rates were 71% and 35% with no significant difference between the two arms. The quality of life and the side effects were equally similar, the same for the progression time (necessary time for getting back to the initial pain threshold). The patients treated with a unique fraction were more often retreated (24% to 6%) but without getting back to the initial pain (26). Data analysis of this survey have been recently published. Excluding the retreatment effect, the unique session and the fractioned pattern remain equal in terms of response rate (27).

Another study including 756 patients compared a session of 8 Gy with 5 sessions of 4 Gy or 10 3 Gy sessions. Three percent of the patients had

---

Figure 1 (*Facing page*) (**A**) Important thoraco-lumbar spine destabilization due to metastatic disease needing preventive fixation to avoid kyphotic evolution or neurological compression. (**B**) Preoperative embolization. (**C, D**) Postoperative X rays and MRI at one-year follow-up. *Abbreviation*: MRI, magnetic resonance imaging.

metastases of unknown primary. The conclusions were identical with the efficiency, and the efficiency duration and side effects were similar in the two arms. The patients treated by a 8 Gy session were more often retreated, but this does not correspond to the upper analogical visual scores (28). Two recent meta-analyses dealt with the efficiency of various radiation patterns. Wu et al. studied the data in eight randomized surveys including more than 3200 patients by comparing a unique 8 to 10 Gy session to various fractioned patterns. The overall response rate and the complete response rate are identical in the two groups (72% and 32%). Similarly, there is no dose effect in the studies comparing various fractioned patterns (29). A review of the Cochrane Database took over the data of 11 randomized surveys including more than 3400 patients. The response rate was also identical regardless of the pattern. The patients treated with a unique fraction needed more often a new antalgic radiotherapy and had a more important fracture rate (3% vs. 1.6%) (30). Therefore, a unique session allows getting an antalgic effect equal to longer patterns, and it allows decreasing the patient movements. However, studies integrating patients' quality of life are necessary. In addition, there are patient groups who need a fractioned treatment using higher doses, such as patients carrying a moderate fracture risk, a medullar compression, or metastases accompanied by an important extension in the soft tissues.

Stereotactic radiotherapy allows a better radiation conformation around the target volume. This treatment may be applied in a unique session or according to a hyperfractioned pattern. The stereotactic radiotherapy in a single session is a treatment used for many years within the secondary cerebral lesions. Here, there are a few data specific to the CUP. A survey reports the results from 15 patients treated for one or many cerebral metastases of unknown primary (31). The Karnofsky performance status was 90 and five patients had secondary extracerebral lesions. An encephalic radiotherapy was associated to 14 patients. The median survival of the 15 patients was 15 months; the median survival of the patients with and without secondary extracerebral lesions were, respectively, 5 and 25 months ($P = 0.04$).

Stereotactic radiotherapy finds new applications in the treatment of secondary extracerebral locations. The main constraint of the extracerebral stereotactic radiotherapy is the need to obtain a precise and reproducible repositioning. The patient's imprecise repositioning is supplemented by the movements related to the organ respirations, such as the lungs or the liver. There are now systems that allow patient repositioning within a 4 mm precision margin according to the three axes (32,33) and most of the authors use 5 mm margins for the planning target volume definition according to the axial directions and 10 mm margins according to longitudinal direction in order to consider the organ movements (34). New respiration-controlled radiotherapy techniques are in the process of evaluation (35). The available clinical results in phase I and II trials mainly consider the treatment of secondary hepatic lesions of digestive cancer. There is no data specific to the metastases of unknown primary. Blomgren et al. team was a pioneer in this field. The applied doses ranged between 15 and 45 Gy, in one to three fractions (36). Herfarth et al. evaluated the feasibility and the results of a single-fractioned stereotactic therapy for 37 patients. Four patients had primary hepatic tumors, 33 hepatic metastases. The applied doses ranged between 14 and 20 Gy at the isocenter, with a minimum PTV coverage per 80% isodose. The tumor size had to be lower than 6 cm, and the number of lesions lower than 4. The local control was 75%, 71% and 67% at 6, 12 and 18 months. No major secondary effect was noticed. Ten patients had anorexia, nausea, or hyperthermia for one to three weeks after the treatment (37). Preliminary results show that a single dose of 20 or 30 Gy in three sessions obtain a local control rate of 75% at one year. There are trials in process dealing with fractionated treatment: an European randomized trial compares a single dose of 28 to 37.5 Gy applied in three sessions; a North American dose escalation trial deals with the toxicity and the efficiency of a hypofractioned pattern (37.5 Gy to 60 Gy in three sessions) (35). This noninvasive technique is designed for nonoperable patients for medical or surgical reasons. However, it is too early to propose it as standard in the local treatment of hepatic metastases.

As we have already seen, there are a few data on secondary lesions of unknown primary related to these various treatment methods. However, new techniques seem to be used on these patients. Radiofrequency is now part of the local treatment of hepatic metastases, while the extracerebral stereotactic radiotherapy should be soon. As far as bone metastases are concerned, a unique radiotherapy session allows getting the same antalgic effect and as durable as the hypofractioned patterns at the cost of a slightly higher fracture risk. Surgery, especially the preventive surgery, may be part of the treatment of these bone lesions. In the future, trials specific to the CUP should be considered in order to better specify the indications and the efficiency of these treatments.

REFERENCES

1. Abbruzzese JL, Lenzi R, Raber MN, Pathak S, Frost P. The biology of unknown primary tumors. Semin Oncol 1993; 20:238–243.
2. Abbruzzesse JL, Abbruzzesse MC, Lenzi R, Hess KR, Raber MN. Analysis of a diagnostic strategy for patients with suspected tumors of unknown origin. J Clin Oncol 1995; 13:2094–2103.
3. Van de Wouw AJ, Janssen–Heijnen ML, Coebergh JW, Hillen HF. Epidemiology of unknown primary tumours; incidence and population–based survival of 1285 patients in Southeast Netherlands, 1984–1992. Eur J Cancer 2002; 38: 409–413.
4. Levi F, Te VC, Erler G, Randimbison L, La Vecchia C. Epidemiology of unknown primary tumours. Eur J Cancer 2002; 38:1810–1812.

5. Chagnon S, Qanadli S, Lacombe P. Percutaneous radiofrequency ablation of liver tumors. Gastroenterol Clin Biol 2001; 25(suppl 4):B85–B99.

6. Curley SA, Marra P, Beaty K, et al. Early and late complications after radiofrequency ablation of malignant liver tumors in 608 patients. Ann Surg 2004; 239(4):450–458.

7. Rhim H, Goldberg SH, Dodd GD. Essential techniques for successful radiofrequency thermal ablation of malignant hepatic tumors. Radiographics 2001; 21:S17–S39.

8. Seifert JK, Morris DL. World survey on the complications of hepatic and prostate cryotherapy. World J Surg 199; 23(2):109–114.

9. Ruers TJ, Joosten J, Jager GJ, Wobbes T. Long-term results of treating hepatic colorectal metastases with cryosurgery. Br J Surg 2001; 88(6):844–849.

10. Goering JD, Mahvi DM, Niederhuber JE, Chicks D, Rikkers LF. Cryoablation and liver resection for noncolorectal liver metastases. Am J Surg 2002; 183(4):384–389.

11. Hawksworth J, Geisinger K, Zagoria R, et al. Surgical and ablative treatment for metastatic adenocarcinoma to the liver from unknown primary tumor. Am Surg 2004; 70(6):512–517.

12. Pavlidis N. Cancer of unknown primary: biological and clinical characteristics. Ann Oncol 2003; 14(suppl 3):11–18.

13. Nakamoto Y, Osman M, Wahl RL. Prevalence and patterns of bone metastases detected with positron emission tomography using F-18 FDG. Clin Nucl Med 2003; 28(4):302–307.

14. Rougraff BT. Evaluation of the patient with carcinoma of unknown origin metastatic to bone. Clin Orthop 2003(suppl 415):S105–S109.

15. Kreder, Hans J. Factors affecting outcome after surgical treatment of acetabular and femoral metastatic lesions. Tech Orthop 2004; 19(1):38–44.

16. Sparkes, J. Upper limb bone metastases. Tech Orthop 2004; 19(1):9–14.

17. Stephen D. Management of metastatic osseous lesions of the lower extremity. Tech Orthop 2004; 19(1):15–24.

18. Wunder JS, Ferguson PC, Griffin AM, Pressman A, Bell RS. Acetabular metastases: planning for reconstruction and review of results. Clin Orthop 2003 (suppl 415):S187–S197.

19. Ratliff J, Cooper P. Metastatic spine tumors. South Med J 2004; 97(3):246–253.

20. Missenard G, Lapresle P, Cote D. Local control after surgical treatment of spinal metastatic disease. Eur Spine J 1996; 5:45–50.

21. Bennet A. The role of biochemical mediators in peripheral nociception and bone pain. Cancer Survey 1988; 7:55–67.

22. Chow E, Danjoux C, Wong R. Palliation of bone metastases: a survey of patterns of practice among Canadian radiation oncologists. Radiother Oncol 2000; 56:305–314.

23. Lievens Y, Kesteloot K, Rijnders A. Differences in palliative radiotherapy for bone metastases within Western European countries. Radiother Oncol 2000; 56:297–303.

24. Chow E, Wong R, Hruby G. Prospective patient-based assesment of effectiveness of palliative radiotherapy for bone metastases. Radiother Oncol 2001; 6:77–82.

25. Ciezki JP, Komurcu S, Macklis RM. Palliative radiotherapy. Semin Oncol 2000; 27:90–93.
26. Steenland E, Leer J, Houwelingen HV. The effect of a single fraction compared to multiple fractions on painful bone metastases: a global analysis of the Dutch Bone Metastasis Study. Radiother Oncol 1999; 52:101–109.
27. Van der Lindem YM, Lok JJ, Steenland E, Martijn H, Houwelingen HV, Marijnen C. Single fraction radiotherapy is efficacious: a further analysis of the Dutch Bone Metastasis Study controlling for the influence of retreatment. Int J Radiat Oncol Biol Phys 2004; 59:528–537.
28. Bone Pain Trial Working Party. 8 Gy single fraction radiotherapy for the treatment of metastatic skeletal pain: randomised comparison with a multifraction schedule over 12 months of patients follow up. Radiother Oncol 1999; 52:111–121.
29. Wu JSY, Wong R, Johnston M. Meta analysis of dose fractionation radiotherapy trials for the palliation of bone metastases. Int J Radiat Oncol Biol Phys 2003; 55:594–605.
30. Palliation of metastatic bone pain: single fraction versus multifraction radiotherapy—a systematic review of the randomised trials. Cochrane Database Syst Review 2004; CD004721.
31. Maesawa S, Kondziolka D, Thompson TP, Flickinger JC, Dade L. Brain metastases in patients with no known primary tumor. Cancer 2000; 89(5): 1095–1101.
32. Herfarth KK, Debus J, Lohr F, et al. Extracranial stereotactic radiation therapy: set-up accuracy of patients treated for liver metastases. Int J Radiat Oncol Biol Phys 2000; 46:329–335.
33. Wulf J, Hadinger U, Oppitz U, Olshausen B, Flentje M. Stereotactic radiotherapy of extracranial targets: CT-simulation and accuracy of treatment in the stereotactic body frame. Radiother Oncol 2000; 57:225–236.
34. Wulf J, Hadinger U, Oppitz U, Thiele W, Flentje M. Impact of reproducibility on tumor dose in stereotactic radiotherapy of targets in the lung and liver. Radiother Oncol 2003; 66:141–150.
35. Fuss M, Thomas CR. New approaches to the treatment of hepatic malignancies stereotactic body radiation therapy: an ablative treatment option for primary and secondary liver tumors. Ann Surg Oncol 2004; 11:130–138.
36. Blomgren H, Lax I, Naslund I, Svanstrom R. Stereotactic high dose fraction radiation therapy of extracranial tumors using an accelerator. Clinical experience of the first thirty-one patients. Acta Oncol 1995; 34:861–870.
37. Herfarth KK, Debus J, Lohr F, et al. Stereotactic single-dose radiation therapy of liver tumors: results of a phase I/II trial. J Clin Oncol 2001; 19:164–170.

14

The Biology of Unknown Primary Tumors: The Little We Know, the Importance of Learning More

Pierre Busson

CNRS UMR 8126, Institut Gustave Roussy, Villejuif, France

Leela Daya-Grosjean

CNRS UPR 2169, Institut Gustave Roussy, Villejuif, France

Nicholas Pavlidis

Department of Medical Oncology, Ioannina University Hospital, Ioannina, Greece

Agnès J. Van de Wouw

Department of Internal Medicine, Slingeland Hospital Doetinchem, The Netherlands

INTRODUCTION

From a biological point of view, two remarkable characteristics attract attention to unknown primary tumors (UPTs): (i) an atypical distribution of the tumor mass between the metastatic and primary lesions, suggesting a relative or absolute inhibition of primary tumor growth and; (ii) a peculiar pattern of metastatic spread with early involvement of multiple organs and rapid progression. Deletions or rearrangements of chromosome 1p and c-myc overexpression are consistently found in UPTs as in other aggressive malignancies. Some other characteristics are more intriguing such as the overexpression of Bcl-2, which is frequent in low grade malignancies but is also frequent in UPTs. There is evidence that p53 is rarely mutated in UPTs. If this is confirmed, this observation could be pivotal in future investigations on the acquisition of the UPT metastatic phenotype. The mechanisms of primary tumor growth inhibition remain completely hypothetical; immune and inflammatory mechanisms might play a role in the inhibition or regression of the primary tumor. New insights on UPT biology will come from high-throughput genome, transcriptome, and proteome analyses. It will be important to combine data on gene expression with data on structural gene alterations. Investigations of p53 and related proteins (p73, Arf, MDM2 etc.) as well as of the Bcl-2 family are among the priorities for a better understanding of the etiology of UPTs.

NOSOLOGICAL CONSIDERATIONS

The definition of carcinomas of UPT is at present based on negative criteria. This term applies to a metastatic malignancy in the absence of an identifiable primary tumor based on clinical examination, and radiological and biological work-up. In essence, a category based on a negative criterion is temporary and committed to be replaced by subcategories based on positive criteria. In current oncology practice, UPT remains a default diagnosis. Each time metastases appear as the predominant signs of a malignant process, the clinical and radiological work-up intends to find a primary tumor. Until recently, this goal was achieved in less than 50% of the cases (1). In some patients where detection of the primary tumor has not been possible during their lifetime, autopsy will disclose primary lesions previously undetected despite thorough radiological investigations. However, there is a consensus that even after autopsy, a substantial proportion of patients remain without detectable primary tumors, therefore forming an inveterate core of "autopsy-negative" UPTs. Depending on the series, their proportion vary from 45% to 16% (2–4). In recent years, there has been a trend to limit sophisticated investigations of patients with occult primary tumors (1). At the same time pathologists have acquired remarkable tools for the immunohistological diagnosis of organ or tissue lineage on biopsy sections of UPT (1). Currently additional new tools for tissue lineage identification are produced by gene expression profiling applied to a series of tumors of known origin. Using this approach, Tothill et al. have built a classifier based on 79 gene markers assessed by quantitative RT–PCR performed on a microfluidics card (low density microarray) (5). This classifier has given encouraging results when tested on a series of 13 UPTs (5). In fact, radiological work-ups, immunohistological or PCR identification of organ lineage, have the same basic aim, which is, whenever possible, to reclassify UPTs in well-known categories of tumors with known primary sites. In current medical oncology practice, this process of reclassification appears essential for the correct choice of a therapeutic protocol.

However, biologists—or clinicians engaged in reflection on UPT biology—tend to have a different approach. They focus on one obvious biological charateristic of UPTs, which is the atypical tumor mass distribution between the primary tumor and the metastases, suggesting a relative or absolute growth inhibition of the primary tumor. To be more explicit, let us consider the three following cases of revealing metastatic syndromes: (i) a metastatic adenocarcinoma without detectable primary and without possible lineage identification by immunohistochemistry; (ii) a metastatic adenocarcinoma without detectable primary but with molecular identification of a colonic lineage (CK7+, CK20−); and (iii) a small asymptomatic colonic adenocarcinoma revealed by large symptomatic metastases. Despite some important differences related to diagnostic and therapeutic procedures, it is tempting to suspect some common biological mechanisms in these three malignant diseases characterized by atypical distribution of the tumor mass. This notion is strengthened by the observation of an unusual pattern of metastatic spread in UPTs. These patients tend to have a larger number of organs involved compared with other metastatic syndromes, with kidney, adrenal gland, skin, and heart being more frequently involved. Remarkably, this atypical pattern of metastatic spread is found both in patients with "autopsy-negative" UPTs and patients with small asymptomatic primary tumors associated with early large metastases. It supports the idea of a continuum between these two entities in terms of genetic and biochemical alterations (2,6). With this in mind, we propose that a reflection is begun on possible novel names for designation of UPT or carcinomas of unknown primary (CUP) syndromes, for example, "early metastatic syndromes with minimal primary tumors" (EMMP) (Fig. 1). We think that an effort of nosological clarification would be useful for the design of future biological studies. For example, instead of planning research projects focused on CUPs, it might be more accurate to include in a unique project all syndromes combining initial metastatic presentation and primary tumors not exceeding millimeters in size, including some metastatic melanoma syndromes.

As a conclusion to these introductory remarks, Figure 1 attempts to classify metastatic syndromes on the basis of tumor mass distribution at the initial diagnosis stage. Classical secondary metastatic syndromes are on one side of the spectrum (Fig. 1); in these diseases, metastatic lesions become detectable several months or years after treatment of the primary tumor (effective or not). The "early metastatic syndromes with concomitant large primary tumors are positioned at the center and finally, EMMP," including "autopsy-negative" UPTs are at the other end of the spectrum.

RESEARCH AIMS AND INSTRUMENTS

The consideration of UPT syndromes (in the rest of the chapter, we will use the term UPT as an equivalent of EMMP) raises questions for both basic and translational research. In terms of basic research, there are two major aims: (i) to determine whether the metastatic phenotype is underpinned by distinct

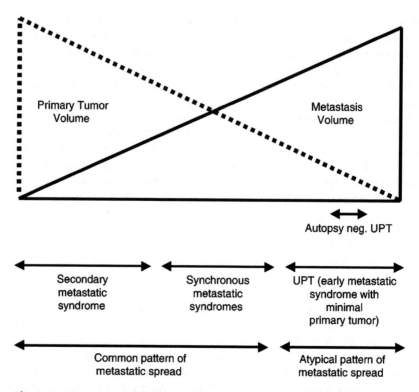

Figure 1 Tentative classification of metastatic syndromes on the basis of tumor mass distribution at initial patient examination. Secondary or metachronous metastatic syndromes are positioned on the left side of the diagram. In these malignancies, metastases are occult at the time of diagnosis and become detectable several months or years after primary tumor treatment. Early metastatic syndrome with minimal primary tumor are positioned on the opposite side. They are usually called UPTs. Initial symptoms result from metastasis development, whereas the primary tumor is asymptomatic or completely occult. Sometimes, it is not even detectable at the autopsy (autopsy negative cases are indicated by a small bidirectional arrow on the very right side of the diagram). Synchronous metastatic syndromes are depicted in the central part of the diagram. At the time of diagnosis and initial evaluation, these patients have clinically apparent metastases and a large primary tumor. Strikingly, early metastatic syndromes with minimal primary tumor often have a peculiar pattern of metastatic spread with simultaneous involvement of several organs, including frequent lesions of the kidney, adrenal gland, skin and heart with rapid progression. *Abbreviation*: UPT, unknown primary tumor. *Source*: From Refs. 1, 6.

genetic or epigenetic alterations in UPTs compared with classical metastatic syndromes and (ii) to elucidate the mechanisms of growth inhibition in the primary tumor. Answers to these questions will bring new insights for our general understanding of human cancers. The most obvious aim of translational research is to contribute to the recognition of clinico-pathological subgroups of UPTs, which can currently benefit from specific treatment modalities or alternatively might become candidates for novel more rational approaches.

There is a critical need for biological resources and laboratory models for biological investigation of UPTs. In addition to potential ethical problems, collection of UPT specimens raises practical difficulties. In the recent experience of the French Study Group for UPTs, specimen collection has been complicated by patient dispersion in multiple medical institutions. When they are referred to specialized cancer centers associated to academic research laboratories, most UPT patients have already undergone tumor biopsy and a significant number of them have already been treated. To our knowledge, there are no studies of animal UPT models with the exception of one report involving the murine bronchoalveolar carcinoma line 1 (7,8). Intravenous injections of these malignant cells in Balb c mice induce pulmonary metastases with concomitant growth inhibition of the same cells when injected subcutaneously. To our knowledge this kind of experiment has not been repeated, but the metastatic properties of the bronchoalveolar carcinoma line 1 is still under investigation as shown by a recent publication (9).

In 1989, Bell et al. reported the establishment and characterization of four cell lines derived from UPTs (10). To our knowledge, these cell lines have not been further studied. One unrelated cell line derived from an adenocarcinoma of unknown primary (metastatic vertebral lesion) has been recently included in the American Type Culture Collection (ATCC; CRL 7431). Thus it would be extremely useful to derive novel in vitro cell lines or stable xenografted tumor lines from clinical samples for biological studies.

BRIEF SUMMARY OF CURRENT KNOWLEDGE ON THE METASTATIC PHENOTYPE

As shown in the previous section, there is a strong suggestion arising from various clinical and pathological observations that UPTs result from specific biological processes which differ, at least in part, from the classical metastatic syndromes. However, published data on biological aspects of UPTs remain rare, even though, there is a huge amount of data derived from classical metastatic models. Therefore, UPT research is naturally and necessarily closely associated with the field of general metastasis research.

The development of a metastatic lesion requires a complex series of molecular and cellular events starting with primary tumor cell release and resulting in invasive growth in a distant organ. This complex process is often called the "metastatic cascade" (11–13). The "successful" metastatic cells have to be able to migrate in tissue adjacent to the primary, cross the vascular barrier, survive in the blood, extravasate in a distant organ, survive in this novel environment, form a dormant micrometastase, and finally be vascularized and escape dormancy. For experimental and conceptual reasons, it is useful to summarize the metastatic cascade as two main phases. The first phase called "tumor cell dissemination" includes all steps from primary tumor release to homing of malignant cells in distant organs. The second phase includes a possible stage of dormancy, the switch to neo-angiogenesis, and finally acquiring the capacity for fully invasive growth (12,13). Owing to the complexity of the metastatic phenotype, it is clear that the metastatic cells have to acquire a wide range of genetic or epigenetic alterations supporting various aspects of their aberrant behavior. Some features of the metastatic phenotype are due to alterations of "metastasis suppressor" genes. For example, there is evidence that silencing of genes like *nm23* or *KAI1* favors tumor cell dissemination by increasing cell motility (14). Other aspects of the metastatic phenotype are caused by uncontrolled expression of metastasis activator genes, such as the genes encoding matrix-metallo-proteinases (MMPs), chemokine-receptors (like CXCR4), or thymosine beta-4 (11,15,16). The MMPs are involved in the increased cell invasion, especially through vascular or epithelial barriers. The chemokine receptors make tumor cells sensitive to chemotactic attraction from a distant organ. Thymosin beta-4 sequesters G-actin and induces dramatic changes in cell morphology and motility.

SPECIFIC AND NONSPECIFIC BIOLOGICAL FEATURES OF UPTs

Pantou et al. have shown that chromosome alterations are, on average, more abundant in UPTs compared with metastases from known primary tumors (17). However, this is not a constant rule. A number of UPTs have only few changes detectable by caryotype examination as well as first generation comparative genomic hybridization (CGH), which is performed on normal human chromosomes used as hybridization substrates (17). In a near future, it will be of major interest to use second-generation high resolution microarray-CGH to investigate such UPTs, which display minimal chromosomal changes according to classical methods (18). Most chromosome alterations reported in UPTs are shared by many aggressive human tumor types, for example losses of 1p and gains of 1q (17,19). Chromosomal gains at 7q22 were reported as frequent potentially specific alterations of UPTs in two independent studies (17,20). There are no clues on which genes are critical for tumor development in this chromosomal region.

The c-myc protein is overexpressed in a large majority of UPTs as in many aggressive human malignancies (21). Surprisingly, Briasoulis et al. have reported overexpression of Bcl-2 in 40% UPTs (22). This was unexpected because in most studies Bcl-2 has been found to be upregulated in pre-malignant lesions rather than in advanced malignancies and has also been associated with a less aggressive phenotype (23,24). To further our insight on this paradoxal expression of Bcl-2, it would be useful to simultaneously investigate the expression of other members of the Bcl-2 family including the pro- and anti-apoptotic members such as Bax and Bcl-X, respectively (25). To our knowledge, there is no information regarding the status of the various metastasis suppressor or activator genes in UPTs, in terms of structure and expression. Investigations of the *nm23* family of genes as well as the MMP, chemokine receptor, and thymosin genes are eagerly awaited.

WHAT IS THE P53 STATUS IN UPTs?

Among the multiple oncogenes and tumor suppressor genes characterized to date, the *p53* gene is the only one for which sequence alterations have been investigated in UPTs. Bar-Eli has reported a frequency of p53 sequence mutations of 26% (6/23) in a series of UPT specimens (15 biopsies and 8 cell lines) (26). This percentage is strikingly low taking into consideration all the data currently available on p53 mutations in carcinomas with a known primary. In the majority of common human carcinomas—including lung, colon, pancreatic, and breast carcinomas—the frequency of p53 mutations is well above 50%, especially at the advanced stages of these diseases (27). In addition, there is evidence that identical p53 mutations are retained in the primary tumor and the metastatic lesions (28). In the study by Bar-Eli et al. it is also reported that a distinct pattern of metastases correlated with the *p53* gene status in UPT lesions (26). Thus patients with wild-type p53 in UPT showed frequent involvement of multiple visceral sites including bone, liver, pleura, and peritoneum. In contrast, the six patients with p53 mutations in the UPT showed primarily lymph node involvement. If the overall low frequency of p53 mutations in UPT lesions is confirmed, it could provide interesting clues regarding the molecular events required for the acquisition of the metastatic phenotype (see next section). A limitation of the Bar-Eli study is that sequence information is confined to exons 5 to 9 of the *p53* gene, whereas it is known that in human cancers, about 20% p53 mutations occur outside this hot-spot region for mutations (27).

More recently, Briasoulis et al. have investigated the abundance of the p53 protein in 47 UPT biopsies by immunohistochemistry (22). A high amount of p53 contained in the malignant cells was found in a majority of patients (53%). As a rule, accumulation of p53 protein is associated with mutations whereas wild-type p53 is rapidly degraded and hardly detectable in tissue sections (29). However, there are several exceptions to this rule. For example, in nasopharyngeal carcinomas (NPC), a malignancy associated with Epstein–Barr virus, which is frequent in southeast Asia and North-Africa, p53 is consistently accumulated in malignant cells despite the lack of gene mutations (30,31). It is postulated that p53 is functionally inactivated in NPC, possibly through the aberrant expression of a truncated form of p63, a protein that has sequence homology with and can bind p53 (32). If it is confirmed that a significant fraction of UPTs show p53 accumulation in the absence of gene mutation, the next step will be to investigate the mechanisms of its functional inactivation. In conclusion, an in-depth re-investigation of the p53 status in UPTs should be a priority. Gene analysis of all 11 exons should be combined with protein detection by immunohisto-chemistry. At the same time, it will be useful to assess the expression of various partners of the p53 network, for example, MDM2 and p19ARF, as well as p53-related proteins p63 and p73, and products of p53 target genes like p21/Waf1 or Bax (33).

ACQUISITION OF THE METASTATIC PHENOTYPE IN UPTs: FROM SPECULATION TO TESTABLE HYPOTHESES

A very important question regarding metastatic syndromes is to know whether the metastatic phenotype pre-exists in the primary tumor or is acquired at various steps of the metastatic cascade through positive selection of additional genetic alterations. The often cited report by Ramaswamy et al. provides strong arguments in favor of the first hypothesis (34). By gene expression profiling of human adenocarcinomas samples of various origin, they have found a 17 gene signature characteristic of the metastatic pheno-type. This signature includes upregulated genes (like small nuclear ribonu-cleoprotein F or securin) and downregulated genes (like actin β2 or the nuclear hormone receptor TR3). Interestingly, this gene expression signature was present in a subset of primary tumors, which were subse-quently identified as being at high risk of metastatic relapse. The authors conclude that in high-risk primary tumors the bulk of malignant cells— and not only a small fraction of them—have acquired the metastatic program. This would explain why even a small primary tumor can exhibit a very strong metastatic potential.

These conclusions have been challenged by more recent studies based mainly on investigation of single, disseminated tumor cells sorted from bone marrow aspirates collected in breast carcinoma patients without clinically apparent metastases. These cells display strikingly heterogeneous chromo-some alterations (35). In addition, they are often p53-negative even when they derive from p53 positive primary tumors (36). This suggests that tumor cell dissemination occurs very early in the evolution of the primary tumor and that disseminated tumor cells subsequently acquire missing pieces of the metastatic program. In this second model, tumor cell dissemination is not only a consequence but also a cause of genetic instability. For example, there is evidence that changes in cell adhesion substrates can induce genetic instability (37). Both models—pre-existing metastatic phenotype or stepwise acquisition—are probably true in some aspects. Interestingly, some reports indicate that p53-mutated primary tumors tend to produce metastases bear-ing the same p53 mutations without additional genetic heterogeneity, in accordance with models postulating a pre-exisiting metastatic genotype and phenotype (28,38). In contrast, metastases derived from wild-type p53 primary lesions acquire a lot of additional genetic alterations although they retain a nonmutated p53. The occurrence of multiple additional genetic changes in the metastatic tissue is consistent with a step-wise acquisition of the metastatic phenotype (28,38).

A priori, both theories of metastasis formation would be compatible with a model of UPT development, provided that the biological mechanisms involved in the relative or absolute inhibition of primary tumor growth are understood. However, if the lack of p53 mutations is confirmed in most UPTs, it will weigh in favor of a stepwise acquisition of the metastatic phenotype. Conversely, a high frequency of p53 mutations or a pattern of gene expression compatible with the 17 gene signature highlighted by Rasmaswamy et al. would be in favor of a pre-existing metastatic phenotype (34).

One additional factor of complexity is that patient's genetic background is believed to modulate tumor cell alterations resulting in the emergence of metastatic cells. In other words, a given type of tumor will not bear the same metastatic risk depending on host genetic background although it is caused by the same initial oncogenic events in various patients (39). This assumption is supported by reports of increased metastatic risks for lung cancer patients carrying specific germ-line polymorphisms of the matrix metalloproteinase 1 (*MMP1*) gene (40). To our knowledge there are no data available regarding germ-line metastasis susceptibility in UPT patients.

THE ENIGMA OF PRIMARY TUMOR GROWTH INHIBITION

One major difference between classical metastatic syndromes and UPTs is the relative or absolute inhibition of the primary tumor growth. This feature remains almost entirely unexplained and it will become increasingly important to address this problem. Several decades ago, Yuhas and Pazmino reported experiments in a murine model suggesting a possible inhibition of primary tumor growth by systemic factors released by metastatic lesions (Fig. 2A) (7). However, in this model as well as in human UPTs, there is no evidence of cross-inhibition between metastatic lesions. One can postulate that the systemic inhibitors released by metastatic lesions have a selective impact on the primary tumor; one possible explanation could be the acquisition of additional genetic or epigenetic alterations underlying the resistance of the metastatic cells to these inhibitors. An alternative hypothesis to explain primary tumor growth inhibition could be through the production of inhibitory factors by normal cells in the microenvironment of the primary tumor (this production would have to be moderate or delayed after an early stage of tumor growth) (Fig. 2B). Metastatic lesions would escape the influence of the inhibitors either because of the distance (for example, if inhibitors are components of the extracellular matrix or are short-lived cytokines) or again because of acquired specific resistance. Human UPT cell

(A)   **(B)**

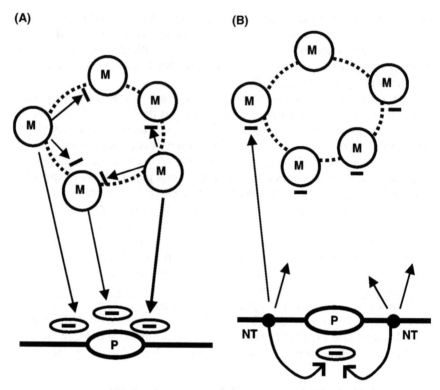

Figure 2 Primary tumor growth inhibition in UPTs: possible action of inhibitory factors. **(A)** In the model proposed by Yuhas and Pasmino, metastatic lesions release diffusible inhibitory factors that block primary tumor growth; implicitly this model postulates that metastatic cells have acquired resistance to the inhibitors that they release (7). **(B)** An alternative model could be the production of inhibitors by normal cells in the microenvironment of the primary tumor (for example, components of the extracellular matrix or labile cytokines). This production would have to be moderate or delayed after an early stage of tumor growth to allow the release of metastatic cells. Metastatic cells would not be reached by these factors or would acquire resistance. *Abbreviations*: M, metastatic lesions; P, primary tumor; NT, normal tissue at the primary site; UPTs, unknown primary tumors.

lines would be useful to address these issues, especially if molecular identification of their primary site can be obtained (for example, using the CK series of antibodies) (1). Then it would be possible to assess their in vitro sensitivity to cytokines known to be produced by their original tissue or organ or even to attempt comparative orthotopic and ectopic xenografts into immunosuppressed mice. The above-mentioned murine broncho-alveolar carcinoma line 1 could also provide a useful experimental system: lung metastases inhibit the growth of a subcutaneous tumor derived from the same cells (7). A good starting experiment to reinvestigate this model would be to make comparative gene expression profiling of lung and subcutaneous lesions.

In the case of "autopsy-negative" UPTs, one needs to assume that the primary tumor has evolved through two distinct phases; a phase 1 characterized by tumor growth allowing the release of metastatic cells and a phase 2 leading to complete regression. Interestingly, rare observations of "burned-out" primary testicular cancers seem to validate such a scenario in the real world of human pathology (41). These patients present with mid-line ectopic germ cell tumors (see next section) whereas attention is drawn to one testicule by detection of calcifications or a notion of cryptorchidism. Orchidectomy and histological examination reveal a fibrous or inflammatory scar, sometimes associated with intratubular germ cell neoplasia. Sometimes an episode of spontaneously resolving gonadal inflammation has been experienced by the patient several months before the symptoms of the metastatic syndrome. In conclusion to their study, the authors suggest that disappearance of the primary tumor might result from an immune response. A higher level of genetic instability in metastatic cells might explain their immune escape. At this point, it is interesting to speculate that inflammation might well be a key process linking primary tumor regression to the development of metastases in UPTs. It is well known that local inflammation is required to achieve tumor regression by immune effectors in both animal models and human pathological conditions (42). On the other hand, some inflammatory cells, especially macrophages, can release cytokines susceptible to enhance cell metastatic behavior and genetic instability, for example CSF1 (43). Therefore, at an early stage of UPT development, inflammation might contribute simultaneously to primary tumor regression and to completion of the metastatic phenotype in a small minority of surviving cells.

SEARCH FOR PROGNOSTIC BIOLOGICAL INDICATORS AND ASSESSMENT OF POTENTIAL MOLECULAR TARGETS

The prognosis of UPTs is extremely severe with a median survival of only eight months. There are well established criteria of bad prognosis including age more than 60, bad perfomance status, liver involvement, and a high level of circulating lactate dehydrogenase (6). So far there have been no additional biological criteria convenient for systematic application in pretherapeutic evaluation. It is worth mentioning, however, that a high microvessel count is an indicator of bad prognosis as is the case in classical metastatic syndromes (44). In contrast, cellular ploidy has no predictive value in UPTs, the prognosis is equally poor for tumors with or without aneuploidy (45). So far, attempts to find additional prognostic indicators by immunohistochemistry have failed. For example, the expression level of CD44v6 or VEGF has no prognostic value (6).

Growth factor receptors with tyrosine-kinase activities—EGF-R, HER2, and c-kit—have recently emerged as promising targets for novel therapeutic agents, especially in some malignancies known to resist all previous therapeutic approaches (46). Therefore, it is important to assess their expression in UPTs. Hainsworth et al. have reported HER2 overexpression in 11% (10/94) of the cases and have proposed evaluation of the efficacy of Trastuzumab in this subset of patients (47). More recently, van de Wouw et al. have found HER2 overexpression in 22% of UPTs (6). However, the proportion of patients with a HER2-positive tumor is much lower (4%, 2/56) in another series investigated by Fizazi et al. [Carcinoma of unknown primary (CUP): are the tyrosine kinase receptors HER-2, EGF-R and c-kit suitable targets for therapy? Manuscript in preparation]. There are no obvious differences in patient distribution between this last series and the two others and it would be probably useful to compare and standardize the staining procedures used by these different groups. A rather low expression of EGF-R and c-kit expression has also been observed by Fizazi et al. (respectively, 4% and 11%).

Proteins involved in the regulation of apoptosis and cell survival are other potential markers of anticancer targeted agents. As mentioned earlier, there is Bcl-2 overexpression in about 40% of UPTs (22). It is noteworthy that taxanes could be used in an anti-Bcl-2 approach. In some experimental models, taxanes prevent polymerization or depolarization of microtubules, therefore inducing phosphorylation of Bcl-2 and resulting in apoptotic cell death (48). Interestingly, in a phase II study paclitaxel has been used in combination therapy in UPTs with promising results (response rates over 40% and median survival of 9–13 months) (49,50).

Apart from the above-mentioned immunohistochemical markers (like CK7, CK20), some cytogenetic markers are useful for improving the recognition of special UPT subsets (1). The best example is the detection of chromosome 12p alterations for identification of testicular germ cell carcinomas without detectable gonadal lesion. This syndrome affects mainly males who are under 50 years of age and is clinically characterized by metastatic disease of a mid-line distribution, usually involving mediastinal and retroperitoneal lymph nodes (1,41). Recognition of the germ cell origin is essential because many tumors of this type respond dramatically to cisplatinum. Cell morphology on tissue sections and detection of serum markers (β-HCG or AFP) are often insufficient for the diagnosis. Because chromosome 12p alterations—iso 12p or 12p chromosome gains—are consistently associated with testicular germ cell tumors, their detection in the context of mid-line UPTs provide both diagnostic and pronostic information (51). Evidence of chromosome 12p alterations substantiate the diagnosis of extragonadal germ cell tumor and predict favorable response to cis-platinum (52,53).

CONCLUSION

Investigation of rare or peculiar malignant diseases have often proved to be useful for our general understanding of cancer biology. Similarly, in the long term, elucidation of some mechanisms of UPT development will probably shed light on more general aspects of metastasis biology, in addition to expected positive repercussions for UPT patients. It is now almost a cliché to say that investigations of UPT will benefit in the near future from genome, transcriptome, and proteome analyses using microarray technologies. One very attractive aspect of microarrays, especially oligonucelotide microarrays, is their capacity to provide simultaneous information on the expression level of a wide range of genes, even using small size clinical samples. It is probably the only approach that will allow rapid sorting of candidate genes critical for UPT development out of hundreds of genes suspected to act as metastasis suppressors or activators. Detection of chromosome gains and losses by microarray CGH will also be of major importance. It is necessary to emphasize the need to combine data obtained from expression and structural gene analysis; for example, it is important to know whether HER2 overexpression in UPTs is associated with gene amplification. Immunohistochemistry will remain essential to validate any information obtained by RNA analysis as well as information from in vitro models or cell lines. We have explained the critical need for additional investigations on the status of p53 and associated proteins as well as on the Bcl-2 protein family in UPTs.

REFERENCES

1. Pavlidis N, Briasoulis E, Hainsworth J, Greco FA. Diagnostic and therapeutic management of cancer of an unknown primary. Eur J Cancer 2003; 39:1990–2005.
2. Nystrom JS, Weiner JM, Heffelfinger-Juttner J, Irwin LE, Bateman JR, Wolf RM. Metastatic and histologic presentations in unknown primary cancer. Semin Oncol 1977; 4:53–58.
3. Le Chevalier T, Cvitkovic E, Caille P, Harvey J, Contesso G, Spielmann M, Rouesse J. Early metastatic cancer of unknown primary origin at presentation. A clinical study of 302 consecutive autopsied patients. Arch Intern Med 1988; 148:2035–2039.
4. Blaszyk H, Hartmann A, Bjornsson J. Cancer of unknown primary: clinico-pathologic correlations. APMIS 2003; 111:1089–1094.
5. Tothill RW, Kowalczyk A, Rischin D, et al. An expression-based site of origin diagnostic method designed for clinical application to cancer of unknown origin. Cancer Res 2005; 65:4031–4040.
6. van de Wouw AJ, Jansen RL, Griffioen AW, Hillen HF. Clinical and immuno-histochemical analysis of patients with unknown primary tumour. A search for prognostic factors in UPT. Anticancer Res 2004; 24:297–301.

7. Yuhas JM, Pazmino NH. Inhibition of subcutaneously growing line 1 carcinomas due to metastatic spread. Cancer Res 1974; 34:2005–2010.

8. Khanna C, Hunter K. Modeling metastasis in vivo. Carcinogenesis 2005; 26:513–523.

9. Andela VB, Schwarz EM, Puzas JE, O'Keefe RJ, Rosier RN. Tumor metastasis and the reciprocal regulation of prometastatic and antimetastatic factors by nuclear factor kappa B. Cancer Res 2000; 60:6557–6562.

10. Bell CW, Pathak S, Frost P. Unknown primary tumors: establishment of cell lines, identification of chromosomal abnormalities, and implications for a second type of tumor progression. Cancer Res 1989; 49:4311–4315.

11. Stetler-Stevenson WG. The role of matrix metalloproteinases in tumor invasion, metastasis, and angiogenesis. Surg Oncol Clin N Am 2001; 10:383–392.

12. Riethmuller G, Klein CA. Early cancer cell dissemination and late metastatic relapse: clinical reflections and biological approaches to the dormancy problem in patients. Semin Cancer Biol 2001; 11:307–311.

13. Pantel K, Brakenhoff RH. Dissecting the metastatic cascade. Nat Rev Cancer 2004; 4:448–456.

14. Yoshida BA, Sokoloff MM, Welch DR, Rinker-Schaeffer CW. Metastasis-suppressor genes: a review and perspective on an emerging field [in process citation]. J Natl Cancer Inst 2000; 92:1717–1730.

15. Muller A, Homey B, Soto H, et al. Involvement of chemokine receptors in breast cancer metastasis. Nature 2001; 410:50–56.

16. Wang WS, Chen PM, Hsiao HL, Wang HS, Liang WY, Su Y. Overexpression of the thymosin beta-4 gene is associated with increased invasion of SW480 colon carcinoma cells and the distant metastasis of human colorectal carcinoma. Oncogene 2004; 23:6666–6671.

17. Pantou D, Tsarouha H, Papadopoulou A, et al. Cytogenetic profile of unknown primary tumors: clues for their pathogenesis and clinical management. Neoplasia 2003; 5:23–31.

18. Pinkel D, Segraves R, Sudar D, et al. High resolution analysis of DNA copy number variation using comparative genomic hybridization to microarrays. Nat Genet 1998; 20:207–211.

19. Abbruzzese JL, Lenzi R, Raber MN, Pathak S, Frost P. The biology of unknown primary tumors. Semin Oncol 1993; 20:238–243.

20. Petersen I, Hidalgo A, Petersen S, et al. Chromosomal imbalances in brain metastases of solid tumors. Brain Pathol 2000; 10:395–401.

21. Pavlidis N, Briassoulis E, Bai M, Fountzilas G, Agnantis N. Overexpression of C-myc, Ras and C-erbB-2 oncoproteins in carcinoma of unknown primary origin. Anticancer Res 1995; 15:2563–2567.

22. Briasoulis E, Tsokos M, Fountzilas G, et al. Bcl2 and p53 protein expression in metastatic carcinoma of unknown primary origin: biological and clinical implications. A Hellenic Co-operative Oncology Group study. Anticancer Res 1998; 18:1907–1914.

23. Pezzella F, Turley H, Kuzu I, et al. Bcl-2 protein in non-small-cell lung carcinoma [see comments]. N Engl J Med 1993; 329:690–694.

24. Kaklamanis L, Savage A, Mortensen N, et al. Early expression of bcl-2 protein in the adenoma-carcinoma sequence of colorectal neoplasia. J Pathol 1996; 179:10–14.

25. Adams JM, Cory S. Life-or-death decisions by the Bcl-2 protein family. Trends Biochem Sci 2001; 26:61–66.
26. Bar-Eli M, Abbruzzese JL, Lee-Jackson D, Frost P. p53 gene mutation spectrum in human unknown primary tumors. Anticancer Res 1993; 13:1619–1623.
27. Hollstein M, Sidransky D, Vogelstein B, Harris CC. p53 mutations in human cancers. Science 1991; 253:49–53.
28. Albanese I, Scibetta AG, Migliavacca M, et al. Heterogeneity within and between primary colorectal carcinomas and matched metastases as revealed by analysis of Ki-ras and p53 mutations. Biochem Biophys Res Commun 2004; 325:784–791.
29. Soong R, Robbins PD, Dix BR, et al. Concordance between p53 protein over-expression and gene mutation in a large series of common human carcinomas. Hum Pathol 1996; 27:1050–1055.
30. Effert P, McCoy R, Abdel-Hamid M, et al. Alterations of the p53 gene in naso-pharyngeal carcinoma. J Virol 1992; 66:3768–3775.
31. Khabir A, Sellami A, Sakka M, et al. Contrasted frequencies of p53 accumulation in the two age groups of North African nasopharyngeal carcinomas. Clin Cancer Res 2000; 6:3932–3936.
32. Crook T, Nicholls JM, Brooks L, O'Nions J, Allday MJ. High level expression of deltaN-p63: a mechanism for the inactivation of p53 in undifferentiated nasopharyngeal carcinoma (NPC)? Oncogene 2000; 19:3439–3444.
33. Benard J, Douc-Rasy S, Ahomadegbe JC. TP53 family members and human cancers. Hum Mutat 2003; 21:182–191.
34. Ramaswamy S, Ross KN, Lander ES, Golub TR. A molecular signature of metastasis in primary solid tumors. Nat Genet 2003; 33:49–54.
35. Klein CA, Blankenstein TJ, Schmidt-Kittler O, et al. Genetic heterogeneity of single disseminated tumour cells in minimal residual cancer. Lancet 2002; 360:683–689.
36. Offner S, Schmaus W, Witter K, et al. p53 gene mutations are not required for early dissemination of cancer cells. Proc Natl Acad Sci USA 1999; 96:6942–6946.
37. Tlsty TD. Cell-adhesion-dependent influences on genomic instability and carcinogenesis. Curr Opin Cell Biol 1998; 10:647–653.
38. Tabor MP, van Houten VM, Kummer JA, et al. Discordance of genetic alterations between primary head and neck tumors and corresponding metastases associated with mutational status of the TP53 gene. Genes Chromosomes Cancer 2002; 33:168–177.
39. Hunter K, Welch DR, Liu ET. Genetic background is an important determinant of metastatic potential. Nat Genet 2003; 34:23–24.
40. Fang S, Jin X, Wang R, et al. Polymorphisms in the MMP1 and MMP3 promoter and non-small cell lung carcinoma in North China. Carcinogenesis 2005; 26:481–486.
41. Fabre E, Jira H, Izard V, et al. 'Burned-out' primary testicular cancer. BJU Int 2004; 94:74–78.
42. Gilboa E. The promise of cancer vaccines. Nat Rev Cancer 2004; 4:401–411.
43. Pollard JW. Tumour-educated macrophages promote tumour progression and metastasis. Nat Rev Cancer 2004; 4:71–78.
44. Hillen HF, Hak LE, Joosten-Achjanie SR, Arends JW. Microvessel density in unknown primary tumors. Int J Cancer 1997; 74:81–85.

45. Hedley DW, Leary JA, Kirsten F. Metastatic adenocarcinoma of unknown primary site: abnormalities of cellular DNA content and survival. Eur J Cancer Clin Oncol 1985; 21:185–189.
46. Sawyers C. Targeted cancer therapy. Nature 2004; 432:294–297.
47. Hainsworth JD, Lennington WJ, Greco FA. Overexpression of Her-2 in patients with poorly differentiated carcinoma or poorly differentiated adenocarcinoma of unknown primary site. J Clin Oncol 2000; 18:632–635.
48. Haldar S, Basu A, Croce CM. Bcl2 is the guardian of microtubule integrity. Cancer Res 1997; 57:229–233.
49. Hainsworth JD, Erland JB, Kalman LA, Schreeder MT, Greco FA. Carcinoma of unknown primary site: treatment with 1-hour paclitaxel, carboplatin, and extended-schedule etoposide. J Clin Oncol 1997; 15:2385–2393.
50. Greco FA, Gray J, Burris HA III, Erland JB, Morrissey LH, Hainsworth JD. Taxane-based chemotherapy for patients with carcinoma of unknown primary site. Cancer J 2001; 7:203–212.
51. Mertens F, Johansson B, Hoglund M, Mitelman F. Chromosomal imbalance maps of malignant solid tumors: a cytogenetic survey of 3185 neoplasms. Cancer Res 1997; 57:2765–2780.
52. Motzer RJ, Rodriguez E, Reuter VE, Bosl GJ, Mazumdar M, Chaganti RS. Molecular and cytogenetic studies in the diagnosis of patients with poorly differentiated carcinomas of unknown primary site. J Clin Oncol 1995; 13: 274–282.
53. Summersgill B, Goker H, Osin P, et al. Establishing germ cell origin of undifferentiated tumors by identifying gain of 12p material using comparative genomic hybridization analysis of paraffin-embedded samples. Diagn Mol Pathol 1998; 7:260–266.

VIII

QUALITY OF LIFE AND PSYCHOSOCIAL ASPECTS

15

Psychosocial Aspects of Cancer of Unknown Primary Site

Renato Lenzi
Department of Gastrointestinal Medical Oncology, The University of Texas M.D. Anderson Cancer Center, Houston, Texas, U.S.A.

Walter F. Baile
Department of Neuro–Oncology, Section of Psychiatry, The University of Texas M.D. Anderson Cancer Center, Houston, Texas, U.S.A.

Chantal Rodary
Department of Public Health, Institut Gustave Roussy, Villejuif, France

Patricia A. Parker
Department of Behavioral Science, The University of Texas M.D. Anderson Cancer Center, Houston, Texas, U.S.A.

INTRODUCTION

Patients with cancer of unknown primary site (CUP) constitute a heterogeneous group with disparate clinical presentations, natural histories, and outcomes. Treatment strategies differ greatly depending on clinico-pathologic characteristics. A few common issues can be identified except for the uncertainty regarding the site of origin of the cancer and a generally unfavorable prognosis with overall survival rates between four months and a year (1,2). A few patients present with isolated lesions that are amenable to local treatment. Approximately 60% of the patients have two or more organ sites involved by metastatic disease (3). The majority of the patients are treated with systemic chemotherapy (2). Some patients with poor performance status (PS) are not candidates for anticancer treatment and receive supportive care only. Survival varies widely for different clinical presentations. Prognostic predictors include PS, number of sites of metastasis, and certain biological parameters [e.g., lactate dehydrogenase (LDH) levels, neuroendocrine histology] (4,5). Long-term survival and cures have been reported in some patients with certain specific presentations, but this represents the exception rather than the rule.

Although there are data strongly supporting the effectiveness of chemotherapy in prolonging survival in certain subgroups of patients with CUP (6,7), whether this benefit extends to the majority of these patients is an issue that has not been resolved. Experience from clinical trials suggests that for patients with presentations including multiple visceral site involvement and adenocarcinoma histology, poor PS, and elevated LDH, chemotherapy is unlikely to favorably affect survival (8,9). Clinical trials formally comparing low toxicity chemotherapy versus best supportive care may provide additional information on this subject (4). Existing evidence has been deemed sufficient by some to issue guidelines recommending supportive care only as the preferred treatment option for patients with PS >2 and other unfavorable prognostic characteristics (10).

Research examining the psychosocial aspects of cancer patients' experience has shown that the negative physical consequences of the cancer and the toxicities related to its treatment are matched in the psychological realm by emotional and social difficulties that place a great deal of emotional stress on patients and families and that can greatly contribute to the deterioration of the patients' quality of life (QOL) (11).

Patients with metastatic disease and poor survival expectations may be faced with multiple challenges including the usually incurable nature of the cancer, the experience of pain, fatigue and functional limitations, the eventual discontinuation of anticancer treatment, and the imminence of death. Although there is some information on the psychosocial characteristics of patients with other types of advanced cancer with known primaries, the psychosocial adjustment and QOL of patients with CUP has received minimal empirical attention. Therefore, there is little specific information available regarding the appropriate intervention strategies to address psychosocial issues in patients with CUP.

While some of what is known about patients with other types of advanced cancer may apply to patients with CUP, there are several characteristics unique to CUP that may influence their psychosocial adjustment and QOL. The CUP patient population is uniquely challenged by the fact that the exact diagnosis is unknown and by the awareness of the fact that the oncologist's recommendations for treatment are not based on the knowledge of the type of cancer they have. As it is commonly expected that physicians proceed to treatment based on a correct diagnosis, the mystery surrounding the type of cancer that is responsible for the patient's condition may add another component of uncertainty to the patient's perception of the illness. Furthermore, the effect of the uncertainty about the diagnosis on the physicians treating these patients is also unknown.

PSYCHOSOCIAL ADJUSTMENT AND CANCER

An emotional reaction to the diagnosis of cancer is normal and expected (12). Commonly, in the first few days after the shock of the initial disclosure of their condition, patients may experience difficulty accepting and coping with the fact that they have cancer and may experience intense hopelessness and skepticism that any treatment will be of help (13) or entertain the possibility that the news may not be true (by using denial or other similar avoidant defense mechanisms) (14). This is usually followed by a period of a few weeks dominated by anxiety, depression, worry about the future, and inability to focus on usual activities. Subsequently, patients often enter a stage of adjustment and coping characterized by the ability to deal with problems realistically, to assess their condition with a more balanced perspective and to concentrate on specific actions (13). Although the majority of patients adjust to their diagnosis and subsequent treatment without experiencing significant distress, there are many who continue to experience high levels of distress and have adjustment difficulties. These may include maladaptive reactions and clinically significant psychological morbidities of varying type, severity, and duration that correlate with a number of factors including pre-existing psychological status, demographic characteristics, physical challenges posed by the illness, and level of family and social support (15).

It has been reported that many cancer patients experience clinical depression, anxiety (16), posttraumatic stress disorder (17), social self isolation, and spiritual/existential crises (15). The construct of psychosocial distress is a useful paradigm encompassing the variety of psychosocial problems described in cancer patients (the most common ones being anxiety, depression, and adjustment disorders) that has been used in numerous studies to characterize the complex illness experience of these patients and to estimate the prevalence of clinically significant psychological and emotional difficulties in this population. The National Comprehensive Cancer Network (NCCN), which is formed by 18 comprehensive cancer centers in North America, established a multidisciplinary distress management panel to define the criteria for diagnosis and management of psychosocial distress. Distress was defined as "a multifactorial, unpleasant experience of an emotional, psychosocial or spiritual nature that interferes with the ability to cope with cancer, its physical symptoms and its treatment. Distress extends along a continuum ranging from normal feelings of vulnerability, sadness and fear to disabling conditions such as clinical depression, anxiety, panic, isolation, and existential or spiritual crisis" (18).

ASSESSMENT AND PREVALENCE OF PSYCHOSOCIAL DISTRESS IN PATIENTS WITH KNOWN PRIMARY CANCERS AND IN PATIENTS WITH CUP

The measured prevalence of psychosocial distress in cancer patients has varied in different studies. Comparisons of these diverse estimates are complicated by the fact that distress has been defined in different ways across studies, the criteria used to define distress levels has varied, and a multitude of measures have been used to assess psychosocial distress. Several factors that affect the prevalence of psychosocial distress including disease-related parameters (e.g., prognosis, stage of disease, and disease burden) (19) and patient characteristics (e.g., age, sex, and socioeconomic status) (15) have been identified. In addition, a variety of instruments have been used to characterize distress that may account for these different estimates. The commonly used instruments have included the Brief Symptom Inventory (BSI) (20), the Center for Epidemiologic Studies—Depression (CES-D) (21), the Hospital Anxiety and Depression Scale (HAD-S) (22), the Profile of Mood States (POMS) (23), and the State Trait Anxiety Inventory (STAI) (24). The corresponding psychometric evidence for each of these instruments has been rated between "excellent" and "moderate" on a five-point scale from "unable to assess" to "excellent" by Carlson et al. (19) (BSI: excellent; CES-D: excellent; HAD-S: excellent; POMS: good; and STAI: moderate).

On the basis of the existing studies, it appears that approximately one-third of cancer patients experience significant levels of distress. For example, in a study of 215 randomly selected cancer patients who were admitted to three cancer centers, Derogatis et al. found that 47% met criteria for a DSM-III diagnosis, with the most common (68%) being adjustment disorders. Anxiety or depression were the main symptoms in 85% of the patients diagnosed with a psychiatric disorder (25). Stefanek et al. studied 126 cancer patients using the BSI, and measured medium to high psychosocial distress levels in 28% (26). In a study of 351 patients with gastrointestinal, breast, urologic, and gynecologic cancers by Parker et al. (27), 32% had CES-D depression scores in the potentially significant range (above the 16 cut-off). The mean overall current anxiety score (STAI-state) was 37.6 for women (corresponding to the 76th percentile compared to a normative sample) and 35.6 in men (corresponding to the 63rd percentile). The study, which also included measures of QOL mental health (SF-12) (28), showed that patients with stage 2 disease reported significantly better mental health QOL than patients with stage 4 disease. Greater perceived social support was also found to be an independent predictor of better QOL in the mental health domain.

Baker et al. (29) studied psychosocial adjustment in 437 cancer patients who were possible candidates for bone marrow transplantation. Thirty-one percent of the patients had evidence of depression (using the

CES-D) and high levels of distress (POMS). Psychological distress was associated with self assessed Karnofsky Performance Status. The incidence of psychosocial morbidity appears to be similar across different cultural backgrounds. Grassi et al. conducted a study of south European cancer patients as part of the Southern European Psychooncology Study (SEPOS) (30). Of a convenience sample of 277 cancer patients studied using the HAD-S, 47 were found to be "clinical cases" on HAD-S Anxiety; 25 were also classified as "clinical cases" on HAD-S Depression. A cut-off score of 11 was used. Forty-seven and forty-four patients, respectively, were classified as borderline case on HAD-S Anxiety and HAD-S Depression with scores 8 to 10, and a total of 34% scored in the clinically significant range for anxiety and 24.9% for depression. A few studies have involved sufficiently large numbers of participants to provide a cross-sectional estimate of the psychological morbidity of patients with specific primary cancers covering a considering spectrum of diagnoses. For example, Carlson et al. examined distress and other psychosocial difficulties in patients with a variety of primary cancers (breast, 23.5%, prostate, 16.9%, colo-rectal, 7.5%, lung, 5.8%, lymphoma, 5.6%, and leukemia, 3.9%). Using the BSI-18 in 2776 patients for whom data were available, 37.8% of patients had clinically significant distress (15). Percentages of patients with distress for the most common diagnoses were 35.4% (breast), 26.6% (prostate), 32.1% (colorectal), 57.5% (lung), 42.5% (lymphoma), and 45.5% (leukemia).

The first report of the prevalence of distress in patients with unknown primary carcinomas is included in the study by Zabora et al. (31) who examined distress in 4496 patients with 14 cancer diagnoses (with no less than 100 patients for each diagnosis). Distress was assessed using the 53 item BSI, consisting of two global scales and nine subscales, with the positive cases being identified based on either a ≥ 63 score on Global Severity Index (GSI) or two of the nine subscales with T-score of ≥ 63 (32).

The prevalence of distress was highest for patients with lung cancer (43.4%) and lowest for patients with ovarian and other gynecological malignancies (29.6%). Of the 129 patients with adenocarcinoma of unknown primary, who comprised 2.9% of the study population, the prevalence of distress was 34.9%. The rates of distress were similar for types of cancer with poor prognosis.

ASPECTS OF PSYCHOSOCIAL ADJUSTMENT IN CUP PATIENTS: ILLNESS UNCERTAINTY, DEPRESSION, ANXIETY, AND PERCEPTION OF PHYSICIAN'S SUPPORTIVE BEHAVIOR

For many cancers of known primary sites, detailed information is available regarding the expected clinical course, treatment alternatives and side effects, probability of response to treatment, and prognosis.

For CUP, clinical presentations are very variable and with the exception of the small percentage of patients who present with well-defined clinico-pathological characteristics, prognostic and therapeutic considerations are difficult to tailor to the individual patient.

For common cancers such as breast, lung, or prostate cancer, extensive information can be accessed by the public through media channels in addition to the information that is available through health care professionals. In contrast, there is little information available to the public on CUP, and for many patients the concept of a malignancy without a defined site of origin is intrinsically difficult to grasp.

A primary factor that is proposed to influence patients' psychosocial adjustment and QOL is the degree of uncertainty regarding diagnosis and treatment decisions. Previous studies about medical illness in general and cancer in particular have identified uncertainty as an important barrier to coping, and greater uncertainty has been associated with increased anxiety and poorer adjustment (33–35). Being diagnosed with CUP would seem likely to generate a great deal of uncertainty in these patients, but to date there has been little examination of this aspect of their illness. Data from a prospective study of psychosocial adjustment in CUP that is ongoing at M.D. Anderson Cancer Center appear to confirm the hypothesis that these patients experience a high level of illness uncertainty. Many of them have symptoms related to psychosocial distress (36). Lenzi et al. examined depressive symptoms (CES-D), anxiety (STAI-state), illness uncertainty (MUIS), and sense of coherence (SOC) in 72 patients with CUP. Demographic characteristics in this sample were consistent with those reported in other studies (sex: 62% male, average age: 59.7 years, married: 86%). The patients had mean CES-D scores of 15.8 [standard deviation (SD) = 10.1], with 41% scoring above the clinical cut-off of 16. The mean score on the STAI was 39.5 (SD = 14.2) with a range of 20 to 70. The mean score on the MUIS was 93.6 (SD = 10.4). In comparison, in a study of lung cancer patients (a population that has been consistently found to experience a high prevalence of psychosocial distress) the mean score on the MUIS was 79.46 (37) and in a study of breast cancer patients the mean score was 76.48 (38).

The behavior of physicians involved in the care of cancer patients can profoundly affect the reactions to the illness, and this is likely to be of particular importance in CUP because of the many unknowns that surround this diagnosis. These patients typically depend heavily on their oncologist for help with decision-making and support. Cancer patients who perceive the physician as caring have been shown to experience lower levels of anxiety (39). In breast cancer, for example, the patient's perception of the physician's interpersonal skills during the diagnostic interview have been shown to be associated with subsequent psychosocial adjustment (40). In a study conducted at M.D. Anderson Cancer Center, Parker et al. studied CUP patients' perceptions of their doctors' supportive behaviors during their initial consultation visit using the Cancer Diagnostic Interview Scale (CDIS) (41), which includes such items as "my doctor understood my fears and concerns" and "my doctor did not take the time to answer all of my questions." Patients' anxiety levels were measured using the STAI. Anxiety was significantly associated with patients' perceptions of their physicians, and the findings suggest that CUP patients who perceive their oncologists as warm, caring, and willing to take the time to provide the information that the patients need experience lower levels of anxiety (42).

QOL INSTRUMENTS IN CUP

In cancer patients, the psychological aspects of their experience of the illness coexist and interact with physical changes that are also related to the illness or its treatment; often their QOL is adversely affected by multiple disturbances in the physical, psychological, spiritual, and social domains with prominent symptoms of distress.

Research in QOL has increasingly focused on the ways in which the experience of cancer exerts its effects on QOL and on the identification of predictors of QOL in cancer patients. This research has highlighted the complexity of the construct of QOL, which integrates physical and psychological variables into a comprehensive assessment of overall health related well being (43–45).

Several instruments have been developed that in addition to assessing parameters relevant to the general population of cancer patients also focus on symptoms and functional problems that are typical or more frequent when certain primary sites are involved. As mentioned earlier, very limited information exists on QOL issues in patients with CUP. Both clinical trials of chemotherapy and natural history studies have largely omitted systematic assessments of QOL, and only very indirect information can be gleaned from those studies that report parameters such as PS that are directly relevant to QOL. Recently, in a step towards the development of systematic assessment of QOL in CUP, Rodary et al. (46) compared patient acceptance of two QOL instruments: the European Organization for Research and Treatment of Cancer QOL Core Questionnaire 30 (EORTC QLQ-30) (47) and a French translation of the Functional Assessment of Chronic Illness Therapy-FACIT (48,49) with adjustment made to the cultural needs of the patient population studied. The sample included 68 patients with CUP. Four indicators of acceptability and the relative preference rate were used for evaluation and comparison of the two questionnaires. Patients had a WHO PS of 0 to 1 and 78% were receiving treatment at the time of the study. An equal number of patients expressed a preference for each instrument. Sixteen patients perceived items from the FACIT as intrusive (related to sex life, worrying about dying, and satisfaction with QOL) and three perceived items from the QLQ-30 as intrusive. Fourteen and five items were considered "difficult" for the FACIT and QLQ-30, respectively. On the basis of the extent of missing data and the number of items the patients regarded as intrusive and unclearly stated, the QLQ-30 was considered to be the preferred questionnaire. However, qualitative analysis of patients' comments suggested that QLQ-30 might better reflect the patients' physical and medical status and the FACIT the patients' perceived existential QOL. As the authors suggested, a new instrument combining these two aspects might be better suited for this patient population (46). Thus, it may be warranted to develop a CUP-specific QOL instrument that addresses the specific issues of this population.

DIAGNOSIS, PROGNOSIS, AND TREATMENT PLAN: PRELIMINARY FINDINGS IN CUP PATIENTS

Numerous barriers exist to the effective exchange of information between physicians and cancer patients, including the intrinsically complex nature of the disease process and treatment, the use of technical terms that are second nature to the physician but often unfamiliar to the patients, and the emotional consequences of dealing with a life-threatening conditions such as fear, anxiety, and depression in both patients and family members. The physician may also experience feelings of guilt and powerlessness, which may affect the interaction. Exchanging information regarding CUP may pose even more of a challenge than in other cancers because of the lack of definitive diagnostic information and incompleteness of the available prognostic data. As part of a comprehensive study of physician–patient communication in CUP conducted at M.D. Anderson Cancer Center, perceptions of oncologists and patients regarding important medical issues were collected immediately after the conclusion of the initial medical interview (50). Patients and their oncologists completed brief questionnaires assessing to what extent the oncologist had discussed topics including the probability of detecting a primary cancer, the probability of the treatment to induce a remission, the probability of survival, and the option of receiving palliative care only. The participants were also asked to provide their estimate of the probability that a primary cancer would be detected, that the treatment would control the cancer, and their expectations regarding survival. Eighty-one patients newly referred with an initial diagnosis of CUP and five oncologists were enrolled in the study. Patients ranged in age from 43 to 86 years, 86% were married, and 69% were males. There was a significant difference between patients and oncologists in their perceptions of the probability of detecting a primary cancer and of the extent to which the expected efficacy of the treatment and the option of palliative care only were discussed. Patients and oncologists did not significantly differ in their perception of the extent to which the probability of detecting a primary was discussed, of the probability of success in keeping the cancer under control, and of the patient's estimated survival. The study highlighted areas of significant differences in the perception of factual information and extent of the discussion between physicians and patients with CUP and suggests the need for interventions aiming at improving the way information is exchanged between physicians and patients.

CHALLENGING PHYSICIAN–PATIENT COMMUNICATION TASKS IN CUP

Breaking Bad News

The majority of oncologists have had no formal training in this difficult communication task, and yet those treating CUP patients will need to perform it frequently. These tasks include disclosing the diagnosis of CUP, informing the patients of treatment toxicities, discussing the lack of curative treatment, and informing patients of disease progression. Performing these tasks effectively requires proficiency in the delivery of bad news. Physicians experience significant psychological difficulty in giving bad news, and some evidence suggests that they may experience the stress of a bad news conversation long after the conclusion of the medical encounter (51). The difficulty with giving bad news has been deemed to originate from the physicians' wish to spare the patient the pain and suffering related to the news and from the physician's own psychological discomfort in giving the news (52,53).

When bad news is given tactfully, honestly, and in a supportive fashion, the patient's experience of the conversation is less stressful. Friedrichsen et al. reported on the patient's perception of "supporting" and "fortifying" of physician's statements conveying the intention of helping the patient through the course of the cancer while sentences such as "there is nothing more to do" were perceived as "abandoning" and meaning that no further support would be provided (54).

Patients who are not informed of the severity of their condition and who have not been provided with opportunities to express their fears and concerns may come to the conclusion that nothing can be done to help them (55), and patients who are told bad news bluntly by a physician who is trying to quickly complete the difficult task of sharing bad news will likely always remember the discussion as cold, frightening, uncaring, and unsupportive. Loge et al. surveyed 497 cancer patients regarding their experience about receiving their cancer diagnosis (56). Significant predictors of patient satisfaction with the conversation included perceiving the physicians as personally interested, being able to understand the information given, being informed in the proper environment (doctor's office), and having more time invested in discussing the information (56). Although the majority of patients wish to have complete and accurate information regarding their condition, some patients feel that the news is forced upon them, unless their right to have the news given according to their preferences is acknowledged by the physician ("are you the type of person who wants to know all the details about his condition?"). Breaking the news of a diagnosis of metastatic cancer means to many oncologists totally destroying the patient's hope and causes them a great deal of discomfort. Often oncologists have a narrower concept of hope than their patients, and tend to equate hope with cure and hopelessness with any outcome short of cure. To patients, reassurance that they will receive the best available treatment, receiving complete information on all treatment option, including those that the physician does not recommend, and being told that the physician will not abandon them are perceived as hopeful (57).

In a study of 351 patients with a variety of different cancers seen at M.D. Anderson Cancer Center by Parker et al. (58), the patients' communication preferences when given bad news of the initial cancer diagnosis or recurrence were elicited. The highest rated elements included: the doctor being up to date on the latest research on the patient's type of cancer, the doctor informing the patient about the best treatment options and taking time to answer all of the patient's questions, the doctor being honest about the severity of the condition, and the doctor using simple and clear language, giving the news directly and giving full attention to the patient. Differences were noted in patients' preferences based on sex, age, and level of education, underlying the importance of tailoring the conduct of the discussion to the individual patient. Cancer type did not predict patients' preferences. Not knowing the primary of origin makes discussing with CUP patients aspects of their condition clearly and understandably particularly difficult. Unless physicians consciously focus on the communication process and use appropriate techniques, it is likely that patients will misunderstand very important facts related to their illness. Thus, patients with CUP may believe that chemotherapy is being given to specifically treat the known metastatic lesions and wonder whether it will affect the (unknown) primary cancer site. Some patients assume that a treatment plan cannot be chosen until a primary cancer is found, and worry throughout the diagnostic evaluation period that they will never receive treatment if none is detected. Some patients believe that it is uncertain whether they have cancer since there is no definite primary site. Much of what patients believe and fear about their condition is not verbalized but nevertheless will affect their reaction and adjustment to the illness. It is important for the physician to elicit the patients' perspective on their condition because many incorrect beliefs can then be clarified to the patient's benefit.

The use of a specific strategy may more reliably result in the oncologist's better understanding and appropriate response to patients' doubts and fears. The SPIKES protocol (59) is a six-step tool that is meant to help the oncologist to achieve the goals of providing the necessary medical information to the patients while helping to create a supportive relationship and facilitating collaborative decision-making. The protocol conforms to consensus recommendations for breaking bad news (60). In the first step (*setting up* the interview) the physician prepares by reviewing the medical information, setting aside appropriate time for the interview with the patient, and deciding with the patient's input who needs to be present. In dealing with CUP, it would be appropriate to prepare to answer questions frequently asked by these patients, such as why the primary cannot be found, whether potentially diagnostic tests have been overlooked, whether the primary will manifest itself later on, and whether the search for the primary should continue throughout the treatment and until one is detected.

The second step (obtaining from the patients their *perception* of the illness) is very important in this patient population because the cryptic nature of CUP easily lends itself to misunderstandings regarding diagnosis and treatment. Simply asking the patients what they have been told about their disease is one way to obtain this information. The third and fourth steps consist of obtaining from the patients an *invitation* to provide the medical information and should include an inquiry into the patient's preferences regarding how the information is handled—very detailed versus more basic information—and of delivering to the patient pertinent medical *knowledge*, using clear language (no medical jargon), and checking for patient understanding. The fifth step consists of addressing the patient's *emotional reactions* to the news; acknowledging the patient's emotions is most of the time all that is needed, and empathic statements are usually the most effective ("I can see how this is difficult for you to hear" or "you seem very sad"). The sixth step consists of outlining a diagnostic or treatment *strategy*, which is usually accompanied by a summary of the action plan.

The SPIKES method allows for tailoring of the medical communication to the individual needs and preferences and its use can help transform an apparently hopeless interaction into an opportunity to support the patient and to strengthen the physician–patient relationship.

Discussing Prognosis

Oncologists are generally reluctant to discuss prognosis in detail with their patients (61), although a solid bioethical foundation exists supporting such discussion, based on the patients' right to receive information that is necessary to make informed decisions. The timing of the discussion is important, since providing the patient with the opportunity to consider prognostic information can been considered a prerequisite for truly informed consent to treatment. Desiring to avoid destroying hope, oncologists may not provide their patients with understandable prognostic information or may disclose partial data only (e.g., estimates of the probability of responding to a certain treatment, but not a survival probability or a survival time frame) (38). Patients may therefore maintain unrealistic positive expectations regarding the course of their illness (62). Some patients may not form a clear idea about the prognostic information provided because they do not have an understanding of the technical terms used (63). Overall, patients have been shown to be unrealistically optimistic when assessing their prognosis (64). An open and clear disclosure of prognostic information could, however, greatly assist the physician and the patient in treatment-related decision-making. Patients are generally more inclined to undergo more aggressive and toxic treatment if they believe they have a good chance to achieve a remission and a significant prolongation of survival, while they may be more inclined to opt for less toxic treatment or supportive care only, if the probability of favorably affecting the course of their illness is minimal. Nuances in the way prognosis is discussed may significantly influence patients' decision-making. Thus, patients who received the same information in a positive context (probability of a favorable outcome rather than probability of an unfavorable outcome) were more likely to choose a more aggressive (and toxic) treatment option (64). In a study by Hagerty et al. (65) conducted on Australia on patients of mostly Anglo-Saxon background, 126 patients diagnosed with incurable metastatic cancer between six weeks and six months at the time of the study completed a questionnaire regarding their preferences for timing, content, and other parameters related to prognostic disclosure. Discussion of survival at the time of diagnosis was preferred by 59% of the patients. A smaller percentage of patients expressed a preference for negotiating the time of the discussion concerning dying (44%) and survival duration (38%). Patients with longer expected survival duration were more likely to prefer having the discussion of prognosis at the time of diagnosis. Verbal description of prognosis was preferred over the use of printed visual representation such as graphs. Not wanting to discuss survival was associated with lower depression scores on HADS. Forty-five percent of the patients wanted prognosis issues to be brought up by the physician.

The prognostic criteria for the majority of CUP patients are not as well defined as for other groups of cancer patients, and while it may be possible in the future to better tailor the formulation of a prognosis to the individual patient (5), only rather broad guidelines are presently available that can be practically applied to the majority of patients. Discussing the known facts regarding the prognosis of CUP patients and sharing the uncertainty involved is a possible approach. However, it is not known what the preferences of CUP patients are regarding sharing of uncertainty by their oncologist. In a study of 216 general medical patients and 46 physicians by Gordon et al. (66), sharing uncertainty correlated with higher patient satisfaction, but was not an independent predictor. Other physicians' behaviors (such as providing more information and fostering a collaborative approach to decision-making) and selection of patients to whom uncertainty was disclosed (better educated and asking more questions) were also associated with higher patient satisfaction, suggesting that a disclosure of physician uncertainty may result in higher patient satisfaction only when other physicians' behaviors accompany it and in a selected population of patients. Additional studies to address this issue in CUP patients are indicated. Cultural considerations play a major role in the formulation of a strategy for the disclosure of prognostic information in cancer. Discussing prognosis in areas of southern Europe or Asia or in ethnic minority communities where diagnosis and prognosis are primarily communicated to patient's families and not universally shared with patients reflects different standards for truth telling than those prevalent in northern Europe, North America, and some other English speaking countries (30,67,68). Attention to cultural differences is conceivably also important when discussing prognostic issues with CUP patients.

In summary, the discussion of prognosis requires from the oncologist an effort to tailor timing, modality of discussion, and amount of information provided to the individual patient. Cultural background, education level, emotional status, and other patients' characteristics that have been shown to affect preferences for prognostic disclosure should be considered (while avoiding stereotyping the individual patient) in planning the discussion of prognosis with CUP patients. It is important to respect the patient's wishes regarding the amount of information desired and the degree of participation in decision-making, and to be mindful that those tend to change with the stage of the illness (69). A similar procedure to that outlined for giving bad news can be used to obtain insight into the individual patient's beliefs and desires for how information should be communicated ("ask before you tell") (59). Care should be taken not to use technical terms that the patient is likely not to understand: lack of the patient's request for clarification may not mean that the patient understands or may be too embarrassed or upset to ask. The physician should be prepared for difficult questions and to follow the patient's lead as to what is important for them to know about; we have observed that several CUP patients have specifically asked what the possible events leading to their death might be, and hesitated to address that issue. However, addressing the question together with providing a plan to minimize any possible pain and suffering has appeared to enhance rather than disrupt their adjustment to the illness.

Discussing Transition to Palliative Care Only

Some CUP patients present with multiple sites of metastasis, prognostically unfavorable metastatic patterns, poor PS, and are too debilitated to tolerate chemotherapy. Other patients reach the same stage after their disease progresses in spite of aggressive anticancer treatment. Unfortunately, the majority of the patients with CUP will need be transitioned to supportive care only. The discussion of such transition can be frightening for patients and families and a source of difficulty and discomfort for the physician.

Maguire et al. have described the use of certain distancing tactics used by health professional involved in the care of dying patients and resulting in the inhibition of patients' expression of their emotional needs (70). Family members may also respond with high levels of distress to certain physician behaviors such as statements that "nothing else can be done," not explaining treatment goals, not providing family members with the opportunity to express their feelings (67). The consequences of communication behaviors on patients' outcome have been reviewed (71). Once again the model described for breaking bad news can be usefully applied: finding out what the patient's perception of their condition is can be invaluable in guiding the physician's communication strategy. Most patients correctly interpret worsening of pain and other symptoms accompanied by increased functional impairment as evidence of progression of the disease and of the inability of anticancer treatment to control disease progression. Most patients are also keenly aware of the negative effects of chemotherapy on their energy level and overall ability to function. Sometimes patients only go along with the recommendation to proceed with additional anticancer treatment in the face of minimal expectations of a positive result out of respect for the oncologist, who may actually have chosen that therapeutic option mainly to protect the patient against the psychological trauma of being told that "nothing more can be done." Exploring the patients' perception of their condition and their preferences for further care can avoid serious misunderstandings, avoid unnecessary/undesired treatment, and provide a roadmap for shared decision-making and appropriate treatment choices. A physician attitude of empathy, truthfulness, attention to avoid projecting an aura of coldness, and lack of interest appears to work best (72). Many physicians find it difficult to help patients maintain realistic hope when the prognosis is very poor, generally because they identify hope solely with cure or remission. It is important to realize that evidence shows that hope is a complex multidimensional construct (73,74) that is not only promoted by the expectation of a favorable medical outcome for the illness but also enhanced by physician behaviors such as regarding the patient as an individual rather than a case, providing information, connecting with the patient (74). In a study of 126 patients with incurable cancer, Hagerty et al. had patients identify physicians' behaviors that they perceived to be hopeful, not hopeful, or neutral (65). Physicians who offered the best available therapy, stated that pain will be controlled and appeared very knowledgeable regarding the patient's cancer were rated as hopeful by 90%, 87%, and 87% of the responders; physician's use of euphemisms (such as using the word growth and not using the word cancer), giving the prognosis to the family first, and appearing "nervous and uncomfortable" were rated hopeful by only 18%, 13%, and 9% of the patients (65). A strategy of setting together with the patient achievable and realistic goals has been recommended as a feasible strategy for fostering hope (75). Examples of realistic goals are success in controlling symptoms such as pain (76), and maintaining the maximum possible level of functioning for the longest possible period of time. Some patients may verbalize unrealistically optimistic expectations regarding the outcome of their condition. It is important to observe their actions before intervening and trying to change their expressed beliefs. While their utterances may sound unrealistic, they may be acting in a way that is appropriate to their situation (putting their affairs in order, mending fences with family members) there is little to be gained from trying to get them to verbalize the understanding that their expected life span is very short. For patients who unequivocally appear to be in denial, a useful technique is to suggest an ambivalent approach. Many patients will respond positively when encouraged to "hope for the best but prepare for the worst" or to "have a Plan B ready."

CONCLUSION

The management of a patient with cancer typically begins with a specific and accurate diagnosis that provides the foundation for treatment decisions. In the absence of an identified primary, CUP patients may feel that the diagnosis is incomplete and that the evaluation may be inadequate, and may believe that their treatment could be optimized and prognosis improved if a primary could be identified. The oncologist may be tempted to order more and more diagnostic tests in the pursuit of the elusive primary. It may help avoid unrealistic feelings of guilt to keep in mind that diagnostic attempts beyond a "complete" (but not unlimited) set of diagnostic tests have been shown to have a very low diagnostic yield, and that the majority of patients presenting with metastatic disease without an obvious primary cancer will be eventually treated without definite identification of the primary site. A longer survival for CUP has been reported in patients initially presenting with a diagnosis of CUP who had their primary detected after additional evaluation (3). Detailed analysis of the determinant of this favorable outcome has shown, however, that the longer survival is limited to patients with specific diagnoses including nonepithelial histology (lymphoma) or certain carcinomas (breast and ovarian cancer) with higher chance of response to chemotherapy (3). For most of the patients with CUP, therefore, the inability to identify a specific epithelial primary probably does not negatively affect response and survival. Although limited data are available to date, current evidence suggests that many patients with CUP experience significant psychosocial distress and it is important for the physician to diagnose, in addition to the physical ailments, and psychosocial distress, since many of its components, such as depression and anxiety, are amenable to pharmacological treatment or psychotherapy. Finally, proficiency in physician–patient communication is an important competency for the oncologists treating patients with CUP, with the potential for improving patient outcomes and to decrease physician's stress.

Ongoing research is being conducted, which prospectively assesses the psychosocial adjustment and QOL of patients with CUP and the associations between illness uncertainty, SOC, religiosity and quality of physician–patient communication, and QOL in patients with CUP. In addition, several ongoing clinical trials in CUP now include a QOL component. The systematic acquisition of knowledge on these aspects of CUP will eventually result in the design of specific interventions aimed at reducing the impact of psychosocial distress and at improving QOL for these patients and will provide evidence-based guidelines for the physicians who are involved in their care.

REFERENCES

1. Nystrom JS, Weiner JM, Heffelfinger-Juttner J, Irwin LE, Bateman JR, Wolf RM. Metastatic and histologic presentations in unknown primary cancer. Semin Oncol 1977; 4(1):53–85.
2. Abbruzzese JL, Abbruzzese MC, Hess KR, Raber MN, Lenzi R, Frost P. Unknown primary carcinoma: natural history and prognostic factors in 657 consecutive patients. J Clin Oncol 1994; 12(6):1272–1280.
3. Abbruzzese JL, Abbruzzese MC, Lenzi R, Hess KR, Raber MN. Analysis of a diagnostic strategy for patients with suspected tumors of unknown origin. J Clin Oncol 1995; 13(8):2094–2103.
4. Culine S, Kramar A, Saghatchian M, et al. Development and validation of a prognostic model to predict the length of survival in patients with carcinomas of an unknown primary site. J Clin Oncol 2002; 20(24):4679–4683.
5. Hess KR, Abbruzzese MC, Lenzi R, Raber MN, Abbruzzese JL. Classification and regression tree analysis of 1000 consecutive patients with unknown primary carcinoma. Clin Cancer Res 1999; 5(11):3403–3410.
6. Hainsworth JD, Johnson DH, Greco FA. Cisplatin-based combination chemotherapy in the treatment of poorly differentiated carcinoma and poorly differentiated adenocarcinoma of unknown primary site: results of a 12-year experience. J Clin Oncol 1992; 10(6):912–922.
7. Ayoub JP, Hess KR, Abbruzzese MC, Lenzi R, Raber MN, Abbruzzese JL. Unknown primary tumors metastatic to liver. J Clin Oncol 1998; 16(6): 2105–2112.
8. Briasoulis E, Kalofonos H, Bafaloukos D, et al. Carboplatin plus paclitaxel in unknown primary carcinoma: a phase II Hellenic Cooperative Oncology Group Study. J Clin Oncol 2000; 18(17):3101–3107.
9. Culine S, Lortholary A, Voigt JJ, et al. Cisplatin in combination with either gemcitabine or irinotecan in carcinomas of unknown primary site: results of a randomized phase II study—trial for the French Study Group on Carcinomas of Unknown Primary (GEFCAPI 01). J Clin Oncol 2003; 21(18):3479–3482.
10. NCCN practice guidelines for occult primary tumors. National Comprehensive Cancer Network. Oncology (Huntingt) 1998; 12(11A):226–309.
11. Dapueto JJ, Servente L, Francolino C, Hahn EA. Determinants of quality of life in patients with cancer. Cancer 2005.

12. Chochinov HM. Depression in cancer patients. Lancet Oncol 2001; 2(8): 499–505.
13. Massie MJ, Holland JC. Consultation and liaison issues in cancer care. Psychiatr Med 1987; 5(4):343–359.
14. Lubinsky MS. Bearing bad news: dealing with the mimics of denial. J Genetic Counsel 1994; 3(1):5–12.
15. Carlson LE, Angen M, Cullum J, et al. High levels of untreated distress and fatigue in cancer patients. Br J Cancer 2004; 90(12):2297–2304.
16. Silberfarb PM, Greer S. Psychological concomitants of cancer: clinical aspects. Am J Psychother 1982; 36(4):470–478.
17. Palmer SC, Kagee A, Coyne JC, DeMichele A. Experience of trauma, distress, and posttraumatic stress disorder among breast cancer patients. Psychosom Med 2004; 66(2):258–264.
18. (NCCN) NCCN. Distress management: Clinical Practice Guidelines. JNCCN 2003; 1:344–374.
19. Carlson LE, Bultz BD. Cancer distress screening. Needs, models, and methods. J Psychosom Res 2003; 55(5):403–409.
20. Derogatis LR, Melisaratos N. The brief symptom inventory: an introductory report. Psychol Med 1983; 13(3):595–605.
21. Radloff L. The CES-D scale: a self-report depression scale for research in the general population. Appl Psychol Meas 1977; 1:385–401.
22. Zigmond A, Snaith R. The hospital anxiety and depression scale. Acta Psychiatr Scand 1983; 67:361–370.
23. McNair D, Lorr M, Droppleman L. EDITS manual for the Profile of Mood States. San Diego (CA): Educational and Industrial Testing Service, 1971.
24. Speilberger C. Manual for the State-Trait Anxiety Inventory: STAI (Form Y). Palo Alto, CA: Consulting Psychologists Press, 1983.
25. Derogatis LR, Morrow GR, Fetting J, et al. The prevalence of psychiatric disorders among cancer patients. JAMA 1983; 249(6):751–775.
26. Stefanek ME, Derogatis LP, Shaw A. Psychological distress among oncology outpatients. Prevalence and severity as measured with the Brief Symptom Inventory. Psychosomatics 1987; 28(10):530–532, 537–539.
27. Parker PA, Baile WF, de Moor C, Cohen L. Psychosocial and demographic predictors of quality of life in a large sample of cancer patients. Psychooncology 2003; 12(2):183–193.
28. Ware J Jr, Kosinski M, Keller SD. A 12-Item Short-Form Health Survey: construction of scales and preliminary tests of reliability and validity. Med Care 1996; 34(3):220–233.
29. Baker F, Marcellus D, Zabora J, Polland A, Jodrey D. Psychological distress among adult patients being evaluated for bone marrow transplantation. Psychosomatics 1997; 38(1):10–19.
30. Grassi L, Travado L, Moncayo FL, Sabato S, Rossi E. Psychosocial morbidity and its correlates in cancer patients of the Mediterranean area: findings from the Southern European Psycho-Oncology Study. J Affect Disord 2004; 83(2–3): 243–248.
31. Zabora J, BrintzenhofeSzoc K, Curbow B, Hooker C, Piantadosi S. The prevalence of psychological distress by cancer site. Psychooncology 2001; 10(1):19–28.

32. Derogatis LR. The Brief System Inventory (BSI): Administration, Scoring and Procedures Manual. 3rd ed. Minneapolis, MN: National Computer Systems, 1993.

33. Landis BJ. Uncertainty, spiritual well-being, and psychosocial adjustment to chronic illness. Issues Ment Health Nurs 1996; 17(3):217–231.

34. Mast ME. Adult uncertainty in illness: a critical review of research. Sch Inq Nurs Pract 1995; 9(1):3–24; discussion 5–9.

35. Molleman E, Krabbendam PJ, Annyas AA, Koops HS, Sleijfer DT, Vermey A. The significance of the doctor–patient relationship in coping with cancer. Soc Sci Med 1984; 18(6):475–480.

36. Lenzi R, Baile WF, Cohen L, Parker P. A study of psychosocial adjustment in patients with metastatic cancer of unknown primary [abstr]. 2004; 13(8): S1–S233.

37. Hsu TH, Lu MS, Tsou TS, Lin CC. The relationship of pain, uncertainty, and hope in Taiwanese lung cancer patients. J Pain Symptom Manage 2003; 26(3):835–842.

38. Hwang R, Ku N, Mao H. Hope and related factors of breast cancer women. J Nurs Res (Taiwan) 1996; 4(1):35–45.

39. Fogarty LA, Curbow BA, Wingard JR, McDonnell K, Somerfield MR. Can 40 seconds of compassion reduce patient anxiety? J Clin Oncol 1999; 17(1): 371–379.

40. Mager WM, Andrykowski MA. Communication in the cancer 'bad news' consultation: patient perceptions and psychological adjustment. Psychooncology 2002; 11(1):35–46.

41. Roberts C, Cox C, Reintgen D, Baile W, Gibertini M. Influence of physician communication on newly diagnosed breast patients' psychologic adjustment and decision-making. Cancer 1994; 74(1):336–341.

42. Parker P, Baile WF, Cohen L, Heads A, Phan L, Lenzi R. Patient's perception of their physicians'communication is associated with level of distress during initial oncology visits [abstr]. Abstracts of the International Conference on Communication in Health Care 2004:1D-04.

43. Campbell A. Subjective measures of well-being. Am Psychol 1976; 31(2):117–124.

44. Bowling A. Health care research: measuring health status. Nurs Pract 1991; 4(4):2–8.

45. Cella DF, Tulsky DS. Quality of life in cancer: definition, purpose, and method of measurement. Cancer Invest 1993; 11(3):327–336.

46. Rodary C, Pezet-Langevin V, Garcia-Acosta S, et al. Patient preference for either the EORTC QLQ-C30 or the FACIT quality of life (QOL) measures: a study performed in patients suffering from carcinoma of an unknown primary site (CUP). Eur J Cancer 2004; 40(4):521–528.

47. Aaronson NK, Ahmedzai S, Bergman B, et al. The European Organization for Research and Treatment of Cancer QLQ-C30: a quality-of-life instrument for use in international clinical trials in oncology. J Natl Cancer Inst 1993; 85(5):365–376.

48. Cella DF, Tulsky DS, Gray G, et al. The Functional Assessment of Cancer Therapy scale: development and validation of the general measure. J Clin Oncol 1993; 11(3):570–579.

49. Lent L, Hahn E, Eremenco S, Webster K, Cella D. Using cross-cultural input to adapt the Functional Assessment of Chronic Illness Therapy (FACIT) scales. Acta Oncol 1999; 38(6):695–702.

50. Parker P, Baile WF, Cohen L, Heads A, Phan L, Lenzi R. Perception of what was discussed during oncology visits: do patients and physicians agree [abstr]? Ann Behav Med 2004; 27(suppl):SO34.

51. Ptacek JT, Fries EA, Eberhardt TL, Ptacek JJ. Breaking bad news to patients: physicians' perceptions of the process. Support Care Cancer 1999; 7(3):113–120.

52. Buckman R. Breaking bad news: why is it still so difficult? Br Med J (Clin Res Ed) 1984; 288(6430):1597–1599.

53. Fallowfield L. Giving sad and bad news. Lancet 1993; 341(8843):476–478.

54. Friedrichsen MJ, Strang PM, Carlsson ME. Cancer patients' interpretations of verbal expressions when given information about ending cancer treatment. Palliat Med 2002; 16(4):323–330.

55. Fallowfield LJ, Jenkins VA, Beveridge HA. Truth may hurt but deceit hurts more: communication in palliative care. Palliat Med 2002; 16(4):297–303.

56. Loge JH, Kaasa S, Hytten K. Disclosing the cancer diagnosis: the patients' experiences. Eur J Cancer 1997; 33(6):878–882.

57. Sardell AN, Trierweiler SJ. Disclosing the cancer diagnosis. Procedures that influence patient hopefulness. Cancer 1993; 72(11):3355–3365.

58. Parker PA, Baile WF, de Moor C, Lenzi R, Kudelka AP, Cohen L. Breaking bad news about cancer: patients' preferences for communication. J Clin Oncol 2001; 19(7):2049–2056.

59. Baile WF, Buckman R, Lenzi R, Glober G, Beale EA, Kudelka AP. SPIKES-A six-step protocol for delivering bad news: application to the patient with cancer. Oncologist 2000; 5(4):302–311.

60. Girgis A, Sanson-Fisher RW. Breaking bad news: consensus guidelines for medical practitioners. J Clin Oncol 1995; 13(9):2449–2456.

61. Links M, Kramer J. Breaking bad news: realistic versus unrealistic hopes. Support Care Cancer 1994; 2(2):91–93.

62. Gattellari M, Voigt KJ, Butow PN, Tattersall MH. When the treatment goal is not cure: are cancer patients equipped to make informed decisions? J Clin Oncol 2002; 20(2):503–513.

63. Lobb EA, Butow PN, Kenny DT, Tattersall MH. Communicating prognosis in early breast cancer: do women understand the language used? Med J Aust 1999; 171(6):290–294.

64. Gattellari M, Butow PN, Tattersall MH, Dunn SM, MacLeod CA. Misunderstanding in cancer patients: why shoot the messenger? Ann Oncol 1999; 10(1):39–46.

65. Hagerty RG, Butow PN, Ellis PM, et al. Communicating with realism and hope: incurable cancer patients' views on the disclosure of prognosis. J Clin Oncol 2005; 23(6):1278–1288.

66. Gordon GH, Joos SK, Byrne J. Physician expressions of uncertainty during patient encounters. Patient Educ Couns 2000; 40(1):59–65.

67. Morita T, Akechi T, Ikenaga M, et al. Communication about the ending of anticancer treatment and transition to palliative care. Ann Oncol 2004; 15(10):1551–1557.

68. Huang X, Butow P, Meiser B, Goldstein D. Attitudes and information needs of Chinese migrant cancer patients and their relatives. Aust NZ J Med 1999; 29(2): 207–213.

69. Butow PN, Maclean M, Dunn SM, Tattersall MH, Boyer MJ. The dynamics of change: cancer patients' preferences for information, involvement and support. Ann Oncol 1997; 8(9):857–863.

70. Maguire P. Barriers to psychological care of the dying. Br Med J (Clin Res Ed) 1985; 291(6510):1711–1713.

71. Ong LM, de Haes JC, Hoos AM, Lammes FB. Doctor–patient communication: a review of the literature. Soc Sci Med 1995; 40(7):903–918.

72. Friedrichsen MJ, Strang PM, Carlsson ME. Breaking bad news in the transition from curative to palliative cancer care—patient's view of the doctor giving the information. Support Care Cancer 2000; 8(6):472–478.

73. Nekolaichuk CL, Jevne RF, Maguire TO. Structuring the meaning of hope in health and illness. Soc Sci Med 1999; 48(5):591–605.

74. Wong-Wylie G, Jevne RF. Patient hope: exploring the interactions between physicians and HIV seropositive individuals. Qualitative Health Res 1997; 7(1):32–56.

75. Von Roenn JH, von Gunten CF. Setting goals to maintain hope. J Clin Oncol 2003; 21(3):570–574.

76. Links M, Kramer J. Breaking bad news: realistic versus unrealistic hopes. Support Care Cancer 1994; 2:91–93.

IX

CLINICAL CASES OF CARCINOMA OF UNKNOWN PRIMARY SITE

CASE 1

A Female Patient with Pleural Extension of an Unknown Primary Carcinoma

Karim Fizazi

Institut Gustave Roussy, Villejuif, France

In November 2001, a 66-year-old woman with no specific medical history was referred for dyspnea and a cough. She was not a smoker. A chest X ray and a computed tomography (CT) scan of the thorax showed right pleural effusion. Clinical examination, including breast and gynecological examination, was normal. The thyroid was mildly enlarged and an ultrasound examination showed cystic lesions. The performance status was 1. A thoracoscopy was performed and it revealed multiple pleural deposits that were biopsied. Pleural liquid was drained to create pleural symphysis. Pathological examination of the pleural biopsy specimens showed involvement by adenocarcinoma, which stained positive for cytokeratin (CK7), thyroid transcription factor (TTF1), and epidermal growth factor receptor (EGF-R), and negative for CK20, c-erbB2, thyroglobulin, and estrogen and progesterone receptors. Serum CA 125 was mildly elevated at 52 U/ mL (normal value <35 U/mL).

Although the pleura was the only detectable tumor site, chemotherapy was decided and started based on the following rationale:

1. The tumor bulk could not be surgically removed or irradiated;
2. the performance status was good;
3. the clinician felt that immunohistochemical findings and the clinical presentation mostly favored a lung or a breast adenocarcinoma, rather than thyroid cancer or another primary.

A cisplatin–gemcitabine regimen was chosen based on the clinico-pathological presentation and also on the results of a recently conducted randomized phase II clinical trial (Culine et al., 2002).

Outcome

This patient received six cycles of cisplatin–gemcitabine, which led to clinical resolution of dyspnea, a radiological response (dry pleura) and normalization of serum CA 125. She experienced cisplatin-related moderate peripheral neuropathy. Chemotherapy was stopped in May 2002. The patient remained progression-free for more than a year. In June 2003, clinical (cough and pain) and radiological pleural progression occurred and that summer, tamoxifen was prescribed rather than second-line chemotherapy. Tamoxifen proved inefficient. She then received docetaxel for disease progression from October 2003 to March 2004; it proved both clinically and radiologically efficient. However, tumor progression resumed in August 2004. The tumor stained positive for EGF-R, and the use of an EGF-R inhibitor was planned but could not be initiated due to aggravation of the patient's clinical status. She finally died in November 2004.

Comment

F. Anthony Greco
Sarah Cannon Research Institute, Nashville, Tennessee, U.S.A.

This 66-year-old woman who developed pulmonary symptoms is found to have a right pleural effusion; pleural involvement by metastatic adenocarcinoma is detected by thorascopy. After a full staging evaluation, no additional sites of cancer involvement are detected. This patient has a well-recognized, but relatively uncommon presentation of unknown primary cancer. This brief commentary will provide some suggestions regarding the clinical and pathologic evaluation of such a patient, as well as the subsequent treatment options.

Following the diagnosis of pleural involvement with metastatic adenocarcinoma in such a patient, several specific clinical possibilities should be considered. Statistically, the most common cause of this presentation is a small peripheral adenocarcinoma of the lung, which involves the pleural surface early in the disease course. In some patients, a peripheral lung lesion becomes apparent on CT scan after drainage of the pleural effusion. This particular patient was a nonsmoker, and therefore was at relatively low risk to develop lung cancer. However, the incidence of adenocarcinoma in female nonsmokers is increasing, and this diagnosis remains a consideration. In such a patient, fiberoptic bronchoscopy would be a reasonable consideration, although of relatively low yield. The second most common cancer to develop pleural involvement in a woman is metastatic breast cancer. Careful breast examination and mammography should be considered. More recently, the magnetic resonance imaging (MRI) scan has demonstrated occult primary breast cancers in a few patients with suspicious clinical presentations.

Subsequent to the time this patient was evaluated and treated, the positron-emission tomography (PET) scan has been recognized to aid in the evaluation of patients with adenocarcinoma of unknown primary site. In this patient, detection of a primary site by PET scanning (reported in 15–25% of unknown primary patients in small series) may have influenced the choice of first-line treatment (1,2).

Specific pathologic considerations in the evaluation of this patient should focus on the diagnosis of the most commonly suspected tumor types. In this patient, the diagnosis of metastatic breast cancer would provide some additional treatment options, particularly if the cancer is hormone-sensitive. Therefore, staining for estrogen receptor, progesterone receptor, and HER-2 overexpression is essential in this situation. A thyroglobulin stain is also reasonable, although the incidence of detecting a metastatic thyroid cancer are small. Otherwise, immunoperoxidase staining and electron microscopy are usually unable to pinpoint the primary site of a metastatic adenocarcinoma. In this patient, the immunohistochemical battery of CK7, CK20, and TTF-1 was performed. Although the pattern of staining (CK7+, CK20−, TTF-1+) suggests a primary lung cancer, it is important to remember that each of these tests has a false-positive and false-negative rate of 20% to 30%, and therefore cannot provide a definitive diagnosis (3).

In this patient, clinical and pathologic evaluation failed to strongly suggest any particular treatable primary site. Therefore, empiric chemotherapy should be the treatment of choice. A number of combination regimens have recently suggested improved efficacy versus older regimens. The combination of cisplatin–gemcitabine chosen in this situation is one of the most active regimens described, and certainly would be an active regimen should the patient have an occult lung or breast primary site (4). Another equally acceptable treatment option would have been a taxane–platinum combination regimen (5).

In passing, it is probably worth mentioning that in some centers a total pleurectomy or peritonectomy is being evaluated for patients with metastatic adenocarcinoma involving only a pleural or peritoneal site (6). This procedure has suggested benefit in patients with mesothelioma, but as of yet, the reports are anecdotal in unknown primary cancers. Although a few long-term survivors have been described, at this point, this approach remains investigational, and certainly this patient was not an excellent candidate due to her age.

This patient actually had a reasonably good response to first-line chemotherapy, with a response duration of more than one year. However, at the time of recurrence, most patients with adenocarcinoma of unknown primary site are difficult to treat effectively. Several agents have demonstrated some activity, including the taxanes, gemcitabine, and 5-fluorouracil. However, response rates to all of these agents are relatively low, and a "standard" treatment is not established. This patient had a meaningful response to docetaxel, which produced symptomatic and objective benefit for six months.

Another currently available treatment option (not available when this patient was treated) is the treatment with an EGF receptor inhibitor. Although there is no published experience with these agents in patients with unknown primary cancer, response rates to these agents have been substantial in nonsmoking female patients with adenocarcinoma of the lung. If this patient indeed has an occult lung primary, she may benefit from such treatment. Further treatment advances in unknown primary cancer will require successful incorporation of novel agents. Therefore, referral of such a patient to a clinical trial, or even a phase I trial with a new agent, would also be reasonable.

References

1. Bohuslavizki KH, Klutmann S, Kroger S, et al. FDG PET detection of unknown primary tumors. J Nucl Med 2000; 41:816.
2. Rades D, Kuhnel G, Wildfang I, et al. Localized disease in cancer of unknown primary (CUP): the value of positron emission tomography (PET) for individual therapeutic management. Ann Oncol 2001; 12:1605.
3. Tot T. Cytokeratins 20 and 7 as biomarkers: usefulness in discriminating primary from metastatic adenocarcinoma. Eur J Cancer 2002; 38:758.
4. Culine S, Lortholary A, Voigt JJ, et al. Cisplatin in combination with either gemcitabine or irinotecan in carcinomas of unknown primary site: results of a randomized phase II study—Trial for the French Study Group on Carcinoma of Unknown Primary (GEFCAPI 01). J Clin Oncol 2003; 21:3479–3482.
5. Greco FA, Gray J, Burris HA, et al. Taxane-based chemotherapy in patients with carcinoma of unknown primary site. Cancer J 2001; 7:203–212.
6. Glehen O, Mithieux F, Osinsky D, et al. Surgery combined with peritonectomy procedures and intraperitoneal chemohypothermia in abdominal cancers with peritoneal carcinomatosis: a phase II study. J Clin Oncol 2003; 21:799–806.

A Favorable Case of CUP with Peritoneal Adenocarcinomatosis

Nicholas Pavlidis
Department of Medical Oncology,
Ioannina University Hospital, Ioannina, Greece

A 62-year-old female, housewife, mother of three children.

Family history	Father died of gastric cancer
Past medical history	Noncontributory
Social history	No history of smoking or alcohol consumption
Present history	A two-month history of abdominal and pelvic discomfort and fatigue
Physical examination	Palpable masses in the abdomen, moderate ascites, and leg edema (right more than left)
Laboratory work-up	Abdominal CT scan revealed enlarged mesenteric and paraortic lymph nodes, peritoneal masses, and presence of ascitic fluid
	Serum CA 125 was increased ($\times 25$)
	FBC, biochemistry, and chest X ray were normal
Surgical laparotomy	Enlarged mesenteric and paraortic lymph nodes compressing the aorta; peritoneal masses up to 5 cm and ascites were found. Uterus and ovaries were normal
Pathology	Biopsy from lymph node and peritoneal mass showed a metastatic, poorly-differentiated adenocarcinoma. Immunohistochemistry was positive for EMA, pancytokeratin, and CA 125,

	and negative for CLA, CEA, LeuM1, CD30; desmin, vimentin, S-100 protein, and PAS
Treatment	She started on chemotherapy with carboplatin and paclitaxel for eight cycles. Abdominal CT scan, clinical picture, and serum CA 125 levels return to normal. She remains disease-free four years later.

Comment

Thierry Lesimple

Clinical Research Unit, Comprehensive Cancer Centre Eugène Marquis, Rennes, France

In this woman presenting with a peritoneal carcinomatosis without ovary involvement and without primary breast or gastrointestinal tumor, the presentation is not in favor of a malignant mesothelioma or a desmoplastic small round-cell tumor (this latter diagnosis would be based upon the young age, undifferentiated histology, immunohistochemistry profile (EMA+, NSE+, Desmin+), and the demonstration of a specific translocation t[11:22]). Thus, the diagnosis is a primary papillary serous carcinoma (PPSC) of the peritoneum.

By analogy with ovarian cancer, the standard treatment of a PPSC consists in an optimal reduction by debulking surgery followed by about six cycles of platin-based polychemotherapy (e.g., a combination of carboplatin and paclitaxel).

Bibliography

Kennedy AW, Markman M, Webster KD, et al. Experience with platinum–paclitaxel chemotherapy in the initial management of papillary serous carcinoma of the peritoneum. Gynecol Oncol 1998; 71:288–290.

Markman M, Kennedy A, Webster K, Peterson G, Kulp B, Belinson J. Combination chemotherapy with carboplatin and docetaxel in the treatment of cancers of the ovary and fallopian tube and primary carcinoma of the peritoneum. J Clin Oncol 2001; 19:1901–1905.

Clear Cell Adenocarcinoma Presenting as a Carcinoma of Unknown Primary Origin

Carmen Balaña, Eva Castellà, and Rafael Rosell
Medical Oncology Service, Institut Català D'Oncologia,
Hospital Germans Trias i Pujol, Barcelona, Spain

An unusual metastatic pattern is typical for carcinoma of unknown primary origin (CUP). In CUP patients whose primary tumor is identified in autopsy, we usually observe a different metastatic pattern than typically found in that site of origin (1). Moreover, CUP syndrome occasionally includes rare histologies whose natural evolution can be different from typical tumors at the same location, as is the case presented here. Immunohistochemistry can more adequately guide the use of examinations to effectively diagnose the tumor origin, avoiding useless explorations, and moreover, it can help identify the most appropriate treatment for a given patient.

Clinical Case

A 66-year-old woman diagnosed with clear cell adenocarcinoma, after a biopsy of retroperitoneal lymph nodes by laparotomy, was referred to our Medical Oncology Service in October 1999. She had been treated in March 1999 for left foot osteomyelitis and myositis, when she experienced a mild worsening of renal function with hypocalcemia, hypomagnesemia, and normal creatinine levels. She was then diagnosed with secondary hyperparathyroidism due to an increased level of PTH hormone, with normal serum 1,25 dihydroxy-vitamin D and 25-hydroxy-vitamin D levels. This alteration was attributed to secondary rhabdomyolysis and renal dysfunction after ruling out other causes of secondary hyperparathyroidism by intestinal biopsy (to rule out malabsorbtion syndrome) and bone marrow biopsy (to rule out lymphoma). A computerized tomography (CT) scan performed to diagnose a tumoral origin showed retroperitoneal lymph nodes of 1 cm in diameter. One month later, toxic syndrome, asthenia, and lumbar bilateral pain started. An increase in the size of these nodes was observed in a new CT scan (Fig. 1A and B), so a laparotomy and a lymph node biopsy were done in September 1999. The final diagnosis was a clear cell adenocarcinoma (Fig. 2).

(A)

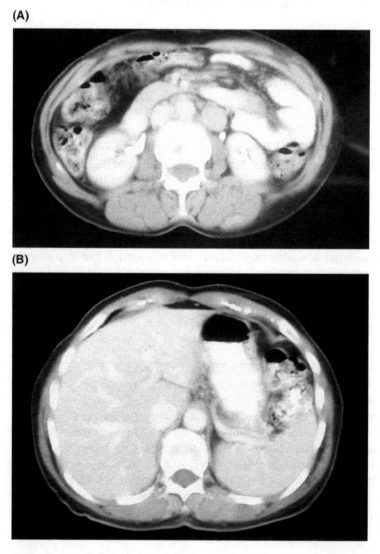

(B)

Figure 1 (A) Retroperitoneal metastasis. (B) Normal liver imaging at the beginning of the disease.

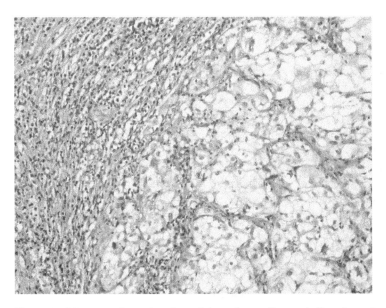

Figure 2   Hematoxylin and eosin staining: clear cell nests infiltrating a lymph node.

Immunohistochemistry with cytokeratines 7 and 20 was not then available at our hospital, and the pathologist recommended we rule out lung, renal and ovarian origins. The patient was sent to our service with a diagnosis of unknown primary carcinoma with retroperitoneal lymph nodes. The only symptoms were a lumbar pain grade 2 and asthenia. Her Karnofsky performance status was 80%. Physical examinations including a gynecological exam were normal. The only alterations detected were anemia, Hb 9.5 gr/dL, with hypocalcemia, 2.13 mm/L (normal value 2.20–2.70 mmol/L) and hypomagnesemia, 0.54 mmol/L (normal value 0.7–1.1 mmol/L), normal phosphorus with increased level of PTH 167 pg/mL (normal values 10–65 pg/mL), and a creatinine clearance of 32.1 mL/min. Tumoral markers CEA, CA19.9, and CEA 15.3 were normal except for CA 125: 64 U/mL. The thorax CT scan and a transvaginal echography were normal. That is, lung, renal, endometrium, and ovary origins, common to clear cell adenocarcinomas, were ruled out by transvaginal echography and CT scans. Positron emission imaging was not an indication for CUP at that time.

As the patient had measurable disease, she began chemotherapy treatment with cisplatin ($70 \, mg/m^2$ day 1, gemcitabine $700 \, mg/m^2$ day 1 and 8, VP16, $700 \, mg/m^2$ day 1 and 2, every 21 days) according to our policy at that time. Calcium and magnesium supplements were administered daily. Doses of cisplatin were reduced to 50% due to creatinine clearance. After four cycles, a normalization of Mg, Ca, and P levels was observed. A CT scan showed a reduction in the size of lymph nodes, and the patient was deemed to be in partial response. She received eight cycles with gastrointestinal toxicity G1.

In April 2000, the lumbar pain reappeared. The CT scan showed an increase in the size of retroperitoneal lymph nodes, as well as in that of the gastric wall. A gastric endoscopy was normal as well as a bone scintigraphy. Calcium and magnesium levels were normal at the time of progression. She began treatment with paclitaxel and carboplatin and completed four cycles. In August 2000, she was admitted to the hospital due to uncontrolled lumbar pain with hemi-abdominal irradiation. Retroperitoneal palliative radiotherapy was administered, and an intrathecal reservoir for morphine was necessary to control the pain. Jaundice and choluria appeared progressively. In the CT scan, a huge mass of retroperitoneal lymph nodes with displacement of pancreas and right renal obstruction was observed; liver metastases and a dilatation of the bile ducts were new findings. (Figs. 3A and B). The patient died on September 9, 2000 and a necropsy was performed.

Results

Necropsy findings showed a clear cell adenocarcinoma with origin in the extrahepatic bile ducts with retroperitoneal metastases, as well as metastases in right kidney, suprarenal gland, ovary, liver, and lung lymphangitis. Immunohistochemistry of the tumor showed a positive immunostaining for CEA++, CK7++ with negativity for CK20. These results confirmed the extrabiliar origin of this neoplasm.

Discussion

Clear cell carcinomas have been observed in kidney, lung, endometrium, and ovary but also in liver, gallbladder, and extrabiliary ducts. Renal cancer is by far the most frequent tumor origin, as the majority of kidney tumors are clear cell adenocarcinomas.

In this case, with CT scans and gynecological exams, we ruled out renal, lung, and ovarian origins—the most frequent sites of this tumor—and we treated the patient with a chemotherapy combination whose activity results have been recently published (2). The patient presented a partial response to treatment that lasted for five months. There was an improvement in her initial symptoms, but within a short period the disease progressed and the patient died with symptoms of uncontrolled retroperitoneal nodes, liver metastases, and a cholestasis. The necropsy found the tumor origin in the extrabiliary ducts.

(A)

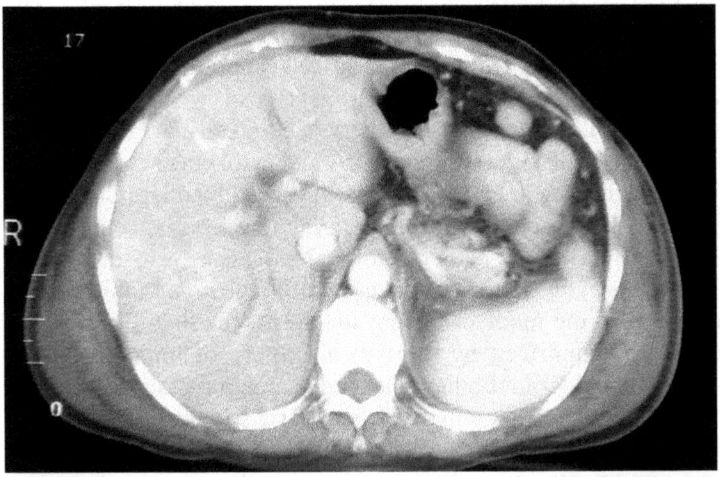

(B)

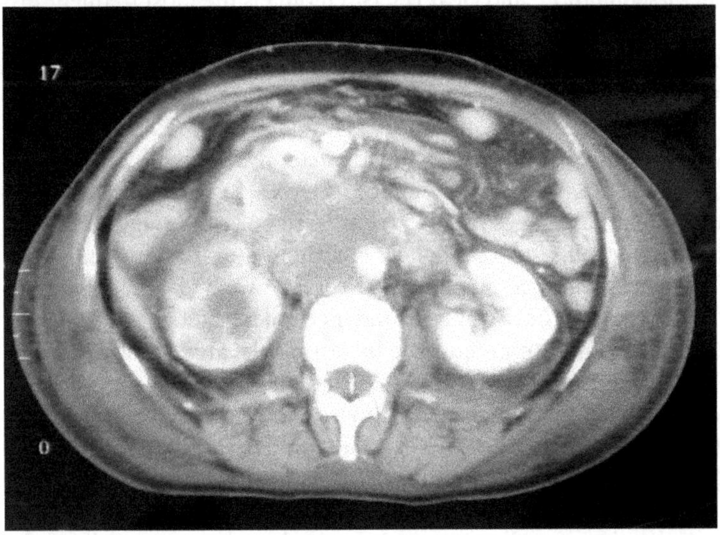

Figure 3 (A) Multiple liver metastases, intrahepatic bile ducts dilatation. (B) Retroperitoneal, renal, and ovarian metastases at the end of the disease.

The majority of malignant epithelial tumors of the gallbladder and extrahepatic bile ducts are adenocarcinomas. Some unusual tumor gallbladder subtypes have been described as signet ring cell, small cell, cribiform, adenocarcinoma with pseudosarcomatous features, undifferentiated carcinoma, and finally, clear cell carcinoma (3).

Tyson and Piney described the first case of clear cell gallbladder adeno-carcinoma in 1926 (4), and he called it hypernephroma due to its similarity with renal cancer. Although infrequent, some reports distinguish clear cell carcinoma of the gallbladder from other clear cell carcinomas coming from kidney, ovary, liver, and endometrium. Bittinger et al. wrote an excellent review on the results of immunohistochemistry of clear cell adenocarcinomas from different origins (5). With the use of CEA and cytokeratines 7 and 20, it is possible to distinguish clear cell carcinoma of the gallbladder (CEA+++, CK7+++, CK20−) from renal clear cell, ovary, and liver clear cell carcinomas (CEA−, CK7− CK20−). Other cytokeratins can help to distinguish between these other origins. In the present case, although immunohistochemistry was not done at the moment of first diagnosis, the final diagnosis of a biliary origin was confirmed by the typical pattern of immunostaining alterations that gallbladder and biliary clear cell carcinomas show.

Although a thoracic-abdominal CT scan and a vaginal echography ruled out lung, ovarian, and kidney origins of the disease, a strong suspicion of renal origin was maintained, as retroperitoneal nodes are one of the first steps of renal dissemination, and clear cell carcinoma is the most frequent histology found in renal cancer. However, the patient was included in a protocol of systemic chemotherapy, as metastatic measurable disease was evaluable in the CT scan and the patient was not a candidate for curative local treatment.

With the necropsy results, the case was re-analyzed. Gallbladder and extrabiliary duct clear cell cancer has already been recognized by the World Health Organization as a separate entity (6). All published cases were females with cholelithiasis, ages ranging from 56 to 68 years. In general, they presented local symptoms such as biliary obstruction and abdominal pain. In spite of the small number of patients, liver involvement, metastases to regional lymph retroperitoneal nodes, and peritoneal metastases have all been reported. CEA and alpha-fetoprotein can be elevated, which was not our case (3,7). No cases of clear cell from the gallbladder or the extrahepatic bile have been reported as a carcinoma of an unknown origin. However, due to the rarity of these tumors (10% of all gallbladder tumors) and the frequency of gallbladder origins in necropsy studies of CUP patients (less than 1%), it must be considered in the case of a clear cell diagnosis. Renal cell carcinoma manifesting initially as a metastatic deposit in the wall of the extrahepatic bile ducts has never been reported and is an extremely rare event (3). Immunohistochemistry can be applied to differentiate among clear cell adenocarcinomas. A cholangio-magnetic resonance imaging (MRI) could have initially been done in order to explore the bile ducts, although the value of this exploration in improving patient prognosis is doubtful, as the patient presented metastases at the time of diagnosis and local treatment would not have been considered. In our case, an adjusted schedule of clinical examinations was undertaken to rule out treatable cancers (8). Positron emission tomography (PET) was not available at that time, although the therapeutic implications of a positive result (abnormal contrast enhancement of the gallbladder) would have had slight impact on the prognosis of this patient.

Recently, gemcitabine has proved useful in the treatment of biliary cancer (9), and perhaps this fact explains the partial response that the patient presented with the schema of chemotherapy she received.

We have found no data on hypocalcemia or hypomagnesemia being associated with a biliary tumor, but a case of a biliary tumor with hypercalcemia and high levels of parathyroid hormone has been recently published (10). In our case, the alteration did not re-appear with the clinical progression, so it is difficult to consider it a paraneoplastic syndrome.

Immunohistochemistry must be done in unknown primary carcinomas to guide the patient diagnosis, and principally to rule out curable cancers and indicate the best treatment to improve prognosis, especially in the metastatic setting of a given patient. However, in spite of most efforts, the prognosis of some patients is not improved as they present metastatic disease, and there is no known useful treatment for the rare entity we diagnose, as in the case of our patient.

References

1. Le Chevalier T, Cvitkovic E, Caille P, et al. Early metastatic cancer of unknown primary origin at presentation: a clinical study of 302 consecutive autopsied patients. Arch Intern Med 1988; 148:2035–2039.
2. Balaña C, Manzano JL, Moreno I, et al. A phase II study of cisplatin, etoposide and gemcitabine in an unfavorable group of patients with carcinoma of unknown primary site. Ann Oncol 2003; 14:1425–1429.
3. Albores-Saavedra J, Molberg K, Henson DE. Unusual malignant epithelial tumors of the gallbladder. Sem Diag Pathol 1996; 13(4):326–338.
4. Tyson W, Piney A. Hypernephroma of the gallbladder. Br J Surg 1926; 13:757–759.
5. Bittinger A, Altekrüger I, Barth P. Clear cell carcinoma of the gallbladder. A histological and inmunohistochemical study. Path Res Prac 1995; 191:1259–1265.
6. Albores-Saavedra J, Henson DE, Sobin LH. The WHO histological classification of tumors of the gallbladder and extrahepatic bile ducts. Cancer 1992; 70:410–414.
7. Vardaman C, Albores-Saavedra J. Clear cell carcinomas of the gallbladder and extrahepatic bile ducts. Am J Surg Pathol 1995; 19(1):91–99.
8. Abbruzzese JL, Abbruzzese MC, Lenzi R, Hess KR, Raber MN. Analysis of a diagnostic strategy for patients with suspected tumors of unknown origin. J Clin Oncol 1995; 13:2094–2103.
9. Scheithauer W. Review of gemcitabine in biliary tract carcinoma. Semin Oncol 2002; 29:40–45.
10. Yen Y, Chu PG, Geng W. Parathyroid hormone-related hypercalemia in cholangiocarcinoma. J Clin Oncol 2004; 22(11):2244–2245.

A Female Patient with a Single-Site Carcinoma of an Unknown Primary Located on the Thoracic Wall

Karim Fizazi and Sylvie Bonvalot
Institut Gustave Roussy, Villejuif, France

A 52-year-old woman with no previous medical history and no smoking history was seen in January 2002 with a tumor of the thoracic wall, located under the left clavicle. Computed tomography (CT) scan and magnetic resonance imaging (MRI) showed that this 7-cm mass was located between the ribs and the pectoralis major (Fig. 1). A biopsy was performed and revealed a poorly-differentiated carcinoma. Surgical resection was performed in April 2002. The pathologic analysis confirmed the diagnosis of a poorly-differentiated carcinoma with positive staining for AEI/AE3 and epithelial membrane antigen (EMA) and negative staining for desmin, chromogranin A, synaptophysin, S100 protein, smooth muscle actin, and cluster of differentiation (CD34).

A complementary immunohistochemical study showed tumor cell positivity for cytokeratin (CK7), and negativity for CK20, thyroid transcription factor (TTF1), estrogen receptors, and progesterone receptors.

A complete physical examination and a whole body CT scan did not show any other detectable lesion nor did a gynecological examination and a pelvic ultrasound examination. A positron-emission tomography (PET) scan was discussed but could not be performed for practical reasons.

The indication for adjuvant radiotherapy to the thoracic wall was not retained because surgical margins were free of tumor. The indication for adjuvant chemotherapy was discussed but finally was not retained.

The patient was regularly followed up by clinical examination and CT scan. She is still relapse-free more than three years after surgery.

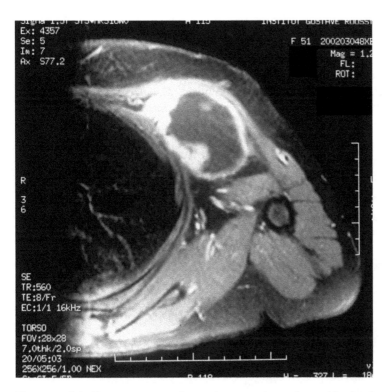

Figure 1 A bulky tumor mass of an unknown primary located in the thoracic wall.

Comment

Nicholas Pavlidis

*Department of Medical Oncology, Ioannina University Hospital,
Ioannina, Greece*

This is an interesting and also an unusual case of carcinoma of unknown primary (CUP). Despite the fact that this 7-cm mass seems an aggressive subtype of CUP, its unusual characteristics are the localized appearance and the three-year disease-free internal without any postoperative therapeutic management. Bronchoscopy findings—although not always necessary in the absence of relevant symptoms or in the presence of an abnormal lung imaging—are lacking. A possible primary origin could be the respiratory system since the tumor was located on the thorax and immunohistochemically was a CK7 positive tumor. This rare case, although characterized as an unfavorable histopathological CUP subset, does at the same time belong to the favorable group of the single isolated potentially resectable CUP tumors. In most of the cases, however, isolated CUP tumors are either squamous cell carninomas or adenocarcinomas in origin. The more than three years disease–free interval is very optimistic, and it is possibly translated to a cured case of a localized highly aggressive carcinoma of unknown site.

Bibliography

Pavlidis N, Merrouche Y. The Importance of Identifying Cancer of Unknown Primary Sub-sets in Cancer of Unknown Primary. In: Fizazi K, ed. (Chapter 4 of this book).

Lesimple T, Balaña C. Carcinoma of Unknown Primary in a Single Site. In: Fizazi K, ed. (Chapter 12 of this book).

Pavlidis N, Briasoulis E, Hainsworth J, Greco FA. Diagnostic and therapeutic management of cancer of an unknown primary. Eur J Cancer 2003; 39:1990–2005.

An Unfavorable Case of CUP with Metastatic Adenocarcinoma to the Liver and Bones

Nicholas Pavlidis

Department of Medical Oncology, Ioannina University Hospital, Ioannina, Greece

A 53-year-old female gynecologist, mother of two children.

Family history	Strong family history of cancer in parents, grand father, and cousins
Past medical history	Chronic pancreatitis–lithiasis since last nine years, cholocystectomy seven years ago. Operated goiter 14 years ago
Social history	Smoker, two packs daily
Present history	A four-month history of anorexia, weakness, and weight loss. One-month history of posterior thoracic pain
Physical examination	Patient almost cachectic, 40 kg, PS 2. A palpable right supraclavicular lymph-node of 2×2 cm. No other abnormalities
Pathology	Biopsy of right supraclavicular lymph-node showed a poorly-differentiated adenocarcinoma. Immunohistochemistry was positive for cytokeratin 7 and CEA, and negative for cytokeratin 20, vimentin, thyroglobulin, P53 oncoprotein, SP-A, and AFP
Laboratory work-up	Liver ultrasound and CT revealed multiple metastatic lesions.

Bone scintigraphy: metastatic sites to thoracic
        spine, ribs, and pelvic bones
Biochemistry: increased γGT($\times$2), ALP($\times$1),
        LDH($\times$1)
Tumor markers: increased CEA($\times$10), CA
        15-3($\times$1), CA 125($\times$50); FBC, chest X ray,
        CT-Thorax, gastroscopy = negative

Treatment   She received combination chemotherapy with
                     carboplatin and gemcitabine as well as local
                     radiotherapy to the thoracic spine. After two
                     cycles liver function tests, tumor markers and
                     abdominal CT showed deterioration.
                     Clinical weekly paclitaxel was given for two
                     weeks without any response. She died four
                     months after diagnosis

Comment

Yacine Merrouche
Institut de Cancérologie de la Loire, Saint Priest en Jarez, France

Unfortunately this 53-year-old colleague presented with common clinical
and histological features of unfavorable subset of CUP. She had a poor
performance status and, multiple liver and bone metastases of a poorly
differentiated adenocarcinoma (1).

Because of the absence of abdominal signs from the immunochemistry
results (cytokeratin 7+, cytokeratin 20−) and of the extrahepatic metastases
we also believe that a gastroscopy was not required (2). Immunohistochemistry staining for TTF-1 (thyroid transcription factor 1) was not performed
but chest CT scan was normal: a pulmonary origin was therefore unlikely.

The disease did not respond to carboplatin–gemcitabine, a regimen
with good tolerability and significant activity in CUP (3). Despite a second-line treatment the patient died rapidly after the diagnosis. This case illus-
trates the poor outcome of unfavorable subset of CUP. In this population an
altered performance status (2 or 3) has been shown to be an independent
adverse prognostic factor (4). In patients with poor-risk disease, low-toxicity
chemotherapy (capecitabine or gemcitabine) is actually challenged with best
supportive care in an ongoing clinical trial (Chapter 10).

References

1. Pavlidis N, Merrouche Y. The importance of identifying cancer of unknown primary sub-sets. In: Karim Fizazi, ed. Carcinomas of Unknown Primary Site. Marcel Dekker Inc.
2. Bugat R, Bataillard A, Lesimple T, et al. Summary of the standards, options and recommandations for the management of patients with carcinoma of unknown primary site. Br J Cancer 2003; 89(suppl 1):S59–S66.
3. Pittman KB, Olver IN, Karapetis CS, et al. Multicenter phase II study of gemcitabine and carboplatin combination therapy for patients with metastatic carcinoma of unknown primary site: final results. J Clin Oncol 2005; 23(suppl 1):8142.
4. Culine S, Kramar A, Saghatchian M, et al. Development and validation of a prognostic model to predict the length of survival in patients with carcinomas of an unknown primary site. J Clin Oncol 2002; 20:4679–4683.

A Favorable Case of CUP with Metastatic Adenocarcinoma of the Liver with Neuroendocrine Differentiation

Nicholas Pavlidis

Department of Medical Oncology, Ioannina University Hospital, Ioannina, Greece

A 75-year old male, father of two.

Family history	Unremarkable
Past medical history	Ten year history of gastric ulcer
Social history	Noncontributory
Present history	One month history of progressive pain over the right hypochondrium
Physical examination	Liver enlargement. Pain on palpation of the right hypochondrium. Rest of PE within normal limits
Pathology	A liver biopsy by computed tomography (CT)-guidance showed a metastatic, poorly-differentiated carcinoma with neuroendocrine differentiation. Immunohistochemistry was positive for epithelial membrane antigen (EMA), pancytokeratin, cytokeratin 8, chromogranin, and neuron-specific enolase.
Laboratory work-up	Ultrasound and CT scan of the abdomen revealed hepatomegaly and multiple liver metastatic lesions Liver function tests showed elevated serum glutamate oxaloacetate transaminase

(SGOT)($\times 2$), serum glutamate pyruvate transaminase (SGPT)($\times 3$), lactate dehydrogenase (LDH)($\times 2$), gamma-glutamyl transpeptidase (GT)($\times 8$), CA19.9($\times 200$), alkaline phosphatase (ALP)($\times 1$)

Tumor markers showed increased carcinoembryonic antigen (CEA)($\times 3$), CA19.9($\times 200$), CA15.3($\times 3$), CA125($\times 23$)

Full blood count (FBC), chest X ray, bone scan, gastroscopy, and colonoscopy were normal

Treatment — Chemotherapy with carboplatin and gemcitabine was started. He received eight cycles every three weeks. He achieved complete remission, which lasted for nine months. He was then treated with weekly paclitaxel for six more months with further partial response. He died 22 months after initial diagnosis

Comment

Stéphane Culine
Centre Val d'Aurelle, Montpellier, France

This is a case dealing with liver metastases revealing a poorly-differentiated carcinoma with neuroendocrine differentiation. I would not have routinely recommended gastroscopy and colonoscopy for this histological subtype because the likelihood of identifying a primary is limited in this setting. Regarding chemotherapy, a cisplatin-based regimen certainly was indicated. I would have recommended a combination of etoposide and cisplatin, but the outcome probably would have been quite similar.

Carcinoma or Melanoma of an Unknown Primary?

Emmanuel Blot and Sophie Laberge-Le-Couteulx
Centre Henri Becquerel, Rouen, France

A 71-year-old woman consulted in January 2002 for left supraclavicular lymph node associated with asthenia. She had no particular previous medical history. Clinical examination was normal except for the presence of left axillary and supraclavicular lymph nodes. The computed tomography scan revealed multiples nodes localized (left supraclavicular region, left axilla, abdominal interaortic-cava, and right inguinal area). Head and neck, oesophagus, gastric, and colonic endoscopies did not reveal any primary tumor. A supraclavicular node biopsy was then performed. It showed an undifferentiated metastasis and the differential diagnosis included carcinoma and a amelanotic melanoma. In immunohistochemistry, metastatic cells were weakly positive for PS100 and vimentin, and negative for a large spectrum cytokeratins (AE1/AE3, kl1, CK7, CK20, CK34 beta E12) and other antibodies against CEA, tumor transcription factor (TTF1), chromogranin, HMB45, CD10, CD68, EMA, and estrogen and progesterone receptors. A cisplatin-based chemotherapy was decided. Clinical and scan evaluation after six cycles showed continued stability of the lymph nodes. Chemotherapy was then stopped. After a 22-month interruption of chemotherapy, the patient remains in an acceptable health status and a very low growth rate for lymph nodes was observed.

Comment

Yacine Merrouche

Institut de Cancérologie de la Loire, Saint Priest en Jarez, France

Pathological examination concluded that standard morphology could be compatible with a carcinoma but that a metastatic achromic melanoma had to be ruled out.

The immunohistochemistry profile was compatible with a melanoma though HMB45 was negative (15% of melanoma being negative for this particular antibody) and a carcinoma far less likely because of the negativity of all cytokeratins and the expression of S-100 protein (6% of undifferentiated carcinoma expressing S-100 protein). A careful dermatological evaluation showed no clinically perceptible presence of melanoma.

A Male Patient with HIV Infection and Carcinoma of an Unknown Primary Site

Roland Bugat

Institut National du Cancer (INCa), Paris, France

A 50-year-old patient was referred to our hospital for right cervical lymph node enlargement. The patient had a 100-pack-year smoking history. He has no history of alcohol or drug abuse. He is HIV positive since 1997 after many journeys in Vietnam and treated by triple therapy antiviral regimen. His CD4 count was 180 mm^3.

He was complaining of exertional dyspnea. Physical exam showed enlarged right cervical, supraclavicular, and axillary lymph nodes, facial and right upper limb edema and thickened and erythematous cutaneous plaques over the neck and right shoulder decreased air entry on both sides, and no hepatosplenomegaly.

1. Which of the following would be indicated in this case?

    a. Complete infectious work-up
    b. Chest X ray
    c. CT scan of neck and thorax
    d. Nasopharyngeal endoscopy

Infectious work-up was negative. Cervical and thoracic computed tomography (CT) scan showed right cervical, supraclavicular, axillary, and mediastinal lymph node enlargement and pericardial and bilateral pleural effusion. No pulmonary lesion. Nasopharyngeal endoscopy showed no suspicious lesion. The biopsy of a cervical lymph node was a poorly-differentiated adenocarcinoma. The patient becomes more dyspneic even at rest. Physical exam shows, in addition to the initial findings, dilated jugular veins.

2. What would be the next step?

    a. Urgent radiation therapy of the neck and mediastinum

    b. High dose of steroids and iv furosemide

    c. CT scan of thorax

    d. Echocardiography

A CT scan of thorax, done to rule out superior vena cava syndrome shows an important pericardial effusion with cardiac tamponade. The patient was transferred to the thoracic surgery unit for urgent pericardiocentesis. Surgical drainage was done with tissue biopsy confirming the previous pathology. One week later, he had a mild dyspnea and was re-admitted to our unit for management.

3. Which one of the following options would be appropriate for this patient?

    a. Cervical and mediastinal radiaton therapy

    b. Chemotherapy

    c. BSC

    d. Oral steroids

He received a combination of cisplatinum (80 mg/m^2 dL) and gemcitabin (1000 mg/m^2 dL, d8 Q 21days). One month later we had a shrinkage of lymph nodes and decreased cutaneous infiltration with no more edema. After three months of treatment CT scan revealed complete disappearance of the bilateral pleural and pericardial effusions with persistent small lymph nodes.

    Thrombocytopenia and neutropenia were the major toxicities and full course chemotherapy could not be delivered on time. Disease progression was the rule but it responds as soon as we resume treatment.

4. What would be the alternative option?

    a. Lowering the dosage of CDDP–gemcitabine

    b. Treatment with monochemotherapeutic agent

    c. Radiation therapy

    d. BSC

    e. Bone marrow aspirate and biopsy

    f. Stopping antiretroviral drugs

Despite lowering the dosage of chemotherapy and discontinuation of antiretroviral therapy, the patient was still neutropenic and thrombocytopenic. We decided to manage the patient with best supportive care. He died five months later.

Comment

A. Plantade, P. Afchain, and C. Louvet
Hôpital Saint Antoine, Paris, France

This case concerns a 50-year-old, HIV positive male smoker with lymph node enlargment and dyspnea. Several pathologies are suspected, particularly infectious and tumoral diseases.

1. Unless the patient presents no fever, opportunistic infectious diseases must be evoked such as pneumocystis carinii pneumonia (dyspnea) and tuberculosis (dyspnea and lymph node enlargment) because of his CD4 account less than 200 mm³. That is why a chest X ray and a complete infectious work-up including a bronchial endoscopy are necessary. A CT scan of neck and thorax has been mandated in order to look for a pulmonary or nasopharyngeal primary carcinoma to investigate all the sus-diaphragmatic lymph nodes, as well as a nasopharyngeal endoscopy. Tobacco use among HIV-infected subjects seem to increase the risk for infectious pneumonia even in case of highly active retroviral therapy. It is also a major risk factor for nasopharyngeal and pulmonary carcinoma.

   Furthermore, some data show that the frequency of lung cancer is increased among HIV-infected patients. HIV infection also increases the risk of AIDS-associated malignancies (non-Hodgkin's lymphoma or Hodgkin's disease).

2. A biopsy of a cervical lymph node reveals a poorly-differentiated carcinoma and since no primary tumor was observed on CT scan of thorax and nasopharyngeal endoscopy, the diagnosis of adenocarcinoma of unknown primary (ACUP) may be retained. In this case the patient presents multiple metastatic sites: lymph node, pericardial, and pleural effusion.

   As the patient is more dyspneic with a right cardiac deficiency, new radiological exams are necessary (CT scan of thorax and echocardiography) in order to eliminate a pulmonary embolism, a thrombosis, or a compression of the superior vena cava.

   High doses of steroids, furosemide, as well as LMWH should not be used in the absence of diagnosis. Radiation therapy of the neck and the mediastinum is not indicated in the case of metastatic adenocarcinoma.

3. After pericardiocentesis, the performance status of the patient is improving. His prognosis remains poor according to prognostic

factors described in several studies (4,5,7). In fact, the patient is more than 35 years old, more than two metastatic sites are involved, and he has a history of smoking of more than 10 pack-years. Nevertheless, platinum-based chemotherapy may be active. In carcinoma of unknown primary, several regimens are used. One of them is cisplatin–gemcitabine combination.

In this case, even if a chest CT scan failed to show a primary lung cancer, a pulmonary origin should be suspected considering the 100 pack-years tobacco story and the localization of metastatic sites. A cisplatin–gemcitabine-based combination fits with this possible diagnosis.

4. A partial response has been achieved after three months of chemotherapy but an important hematotoxicity reduces dose-intensity. Most often, hematotoxicity is caused both by active antiretroviral therapy and chemotherapy. Since a partial response is achieved, best supportive care is not suggested. In this case, antiretroviral therapy should be stopped for a while. The dose of chemotherapy needs to be reduced too. No randomized study has compared first-line therapy the activity of cisplatin as single-agent to the cisplatin-based combination. Lowering the dose of both gemcitabine and platin is a possibility but the activity of both drugs may be reduced. Another possibility is to use cisplatin as a single-agent without lowering its dose.

References

1. Miguez-Burbano MJ, Ashkin D, Rodriguez A, et al. Increased risk of Pneumocystis carinii and community-acquired pneumonia with tobacco use in HIV disease. Int J Infect Dis 2005.
2. Dufour V, Cadranel J, Wislez M, et al. Changes in the pattern of respiratory diseases necessitating hospitalization of HIV-infected patients since the advent of highly active antiretroviral therapy. Lung 2004; 182(6):331–341.
3. Lim ST, Levine AM. Non-AIDS-defining cancers and HIV infection. Curr Infect Dis Rep 2005; 7(3):227–234.
4. Hainsworth JD, Johnson DH, Greco FA. Cisplatin-based combination chemotherapy in the treatment of poorly differentiated carcinoma and poorly differentiated adenocarcinoma of unknown primary site: results of a 12-year experience. J Clin Oncol 1992; 10(6):912–922.
5. Lenzi R, Hess KR, Abbruzzese MC, Raber MN, Ordonez NG, Abbruzzese JL. Poorly differentiated carcinoma and poorly differentiated adenocarcinoma of unknown origin: favorable subsets of patients with unknown-primary carcinoma? J Clin Oncol 1997; 15(5):2056–2066.

6. Schiller JH, Harrington D, Belani CP, et al. Eastern Cooperative Oncology Group. Comparison of four chemotherapy regimens for advanced non-small-cell lung cancer. N Engl J Med 2002; 346(2):92–98.
7. van der Gaast A, Verweij J, Planting AS, Hop WC, Stoter G. Simple prognostic model to predict survival in patients with undifferentiated carcinoma of unknown primary site. J Clin Oncol 1995; 13(7):1720–1725.

A 66-Year-Old Male with Liver Metastases of an Unknown Primary Site

Roland Bugat

Institut National du Cancer (INCa), Paris, France

This is a 66-year-old male patient referred to our hospital for fatigue and loss of weight. On past medical history, he had a diabetes and a myocardial infarction 10 years before. One month prior to consultation, he noticed progressive fatigue and loss of weight (7 kg in one month) with mild loss of appetite. He did not complain of other symptoms, no abdominal pain, diarrhea or constipation, no melena or hematochezia.

On physical examination, he had a PS WHO score 1; he was mildly icteric with no cardiopumonary abnormalities. He had a hepatomegaly 4 cm below the right costal margin firm and nontender, no palpable peripheral lymph nodes and no testicular mass. Digital rectal exam showed normal prostate gland with no suspicious nodule.

1. Which of the following exams would be indicated?
   a. Gastroscopy and/or colonoscopy
   b. Laboratory tests
   c. Chest X ray
   d. Liver ultrasoud
   e. Computed tomography (CT) scan of abdomen

On laboratory tests, CBCD was unremarkable but liver function tests showed both cholestatic and cytolytic abnormalities. Chest X ray was normal.

On abdomino-pelvic CT scan, the hepatic parenchyma was heterogenous, full of multiple small nodules, a 1 cm splenic nodule and a celiac adenopathy were also seen.

2. What would be your next step?

    a. Gastroscopy and/or colonoscopy
    b. CT scan of thorax
    c. Ultrasound-guided liver biopsy
    d. Bone scan

A U/S-guided percutaneous liver biopsy was done. Pathological examination showed a well-differentiated adenocarcinoma that stained positive for EMA, cytokeratin (CK7), CK20, and CEA and negative for PSA and tumor transcription factor (TTF-1).

3. What therapeutic option would you suggest?

    a. Irradiation of the abdomen wall
    b. Cisplatin-based chemotherapy
    c. Single agent chemotherapy
    d. Best supportive care

We decided to treat him with an association of carboplatin–gemcitabine (carboplatin AUC 4 d1 and gemcitabine $1000 \, mg/m^2$ dL, d8 Q21days).

After two cycles of chemotherapy, the disease kept on progressing, the patient had a PS WHO score 3; he was icteric and complaining of diffuse abdominal pain and ascites.

We discontinued all cytotoxic treatment and proceeded to palliative care. The patient died one month later.

Comment

A. Plantade, P. Afchain, and C. Louvet
Hôpital Saint Antoine, Paris, France

This case reports a 66-year-old man who complains of loss of weight and asthenia. Clinical exam shows hepatomegaly with icter. A malignancy is suspected.

1. Laboratory tests are useful to evaluate liver and renal functions, blood cells count, to search for an inflammatory syndrome. An abdominal CT scan is necessary to explore the whole abdominal cavity, particularly the liver and the bladder, as well as the retroperitoneum. The liver ultrasound is of no interest if CT scan is performed.

A chest X ray is recommended in order to rule out pulmonary lesions (metastasis or primary malignancy).

2. Diffuse liver metastasis, a splenic nodule and a coeliac adenopathy have been seen on CT scan. Since colorectal cancer is one of the most frequent neoplasm, especially in case of liver metastasis, a coloscopy is required. If there is no colonic lesion, the next step is the ultrasound-guided liver biopsy. Waiting for the pathological results, a CT scan of thorax and a bone scan may be performed but are not useful for diagnosis.

3. A well-differentiated adenocarcinoma (EMA and CEA positive) has been diagnosed on liver biopsy. Diagnostic investigations failed to show the primary cancer. In this case, immunochemistry test using a specific antibody batter should be performed for the histopathologic diagnosis. It may be very helpful to find out the primary cancer. A digestive origin is possible since CK7 and CK20 are positive. A pulmonary origin is not likely (TTF-1 is negative) as well as a prostatic origin (PSA is negative). In case of liver involvement, neuroendocrine stainings (NSE, chromogranin, and synaptophysin) are requested. In fact the aim of the diagnosis is to identify specific anatomoclinical forms that can be treated by a specific treatment.

In this case, clinical (hepatomegaly with icter), radiological (liver metastases with a celiac adenopathy), and immunochemical (positivity of cytokeratin 7 and 20) findings are in favor of a digestive primary especially a pancreatic one. In case of hepatic and abdominal lymph node metastases, carcinoma of unknown primary are most often occult pancreatic cancers. Abdominal radiation therapy does not make sense because the liver is involved. The performance status of the patient fits with a treatment. A platinum-based chemotherapy should be recommended. Even if a bitherapy never showed significant increase of survival a combination of platin and gemcitabine could be recommended in case of pancreatic origin. Here the choice for carboplatin, which has no nephrotoxicity and does not request hyperhydration, is adapted to the past medical exam of the patient (diabetes mellitus and heavy cardiac history). Gemcitabine–oxaliplatin regimen could be discussed considering the activity of oxaliplatin on digestive cancers.

Bibliography

Bugat R, Bataillard A, Lesimple T, et al. FNCLCC. Summary of the Standards, Options and Recommendations for the management of patients with carcinoma of unknown primary site (2002). Br J Cancer 2003; 89(suppl 1):S59–S66.

Ayoub JP, Hess KR, Abbruzzese MC, Lenzi R, Raber MN, Abbruzzese JL. Unknown primary tumors metastatic to liver. J Clin Oncol 1998; 16(6): 2105–2112.

Tot T, Samii S. The clinical relevance of cytokeratin phenotyping in needle biopsy of liver metastasis. APMIS 2003; 111(12):1075–1082.

Tot T. Adenocarcinomas metastatic to the liver: the value of cytokeratins 20 and 7 in the search for unknown primary tumors. Cancer 1999; 85(1):171–177.

Abbruzzese JL, Abbruzzese MC, Hess KR, Raber MN, Lenzi R, Frost P. Unknown primary carcinoma: natural history and prognostic factors in 657 consecutive patients. J Clin Oncol 1994; 12(6):1272–1280.

Saghatchian M, Fizazi K, Borel C, et al. Carcinoma of an unknown primary site: a chemotherapy strategy based on histological differentiation—results of a prospective study. Ann Oncol 2001; 12(4):535–540.

Louvet C, Labianca R, Hammel P, et al. GERCOR; GISCAD. Gemcitabine in combination with oxaliplatin compared with gemcitabine alone in locally advanced or metastatic pancreatic cancer: results of a GERCOR and GISCAD phase III trial. J Clin Oncol 2005; 23(15):3509–3516.

An Undifferentiated Carcinoma of an Unknown Primary of the Middle Line in a Young Adult

Roland Bugat

Institut National du Cancer (INCa), Paris, France

A 21-year-old patient presents with multiple left cervical and supraclavicular enlarged lymph nodes. He has no complaints, no dysphagia, odynophagia, respiratory, digestive, or systemic symptoms. He has been previously healthy with no past medical history, no tobacco or alcohol abuse.

Physical exam shows multiple enlarged left cervical and supraclavicular lymph nodes, a palpable mass in the right iliac fossa, and the remainder of the exam is negative.

1. What would you recommend as the next step for this patient?

    a. Excisional biopsy
    b. Gastroscopy and/or colonoscopy
    c. Computed tomography (CT) scan of the chest, abdomen, and pelvis
    d. Biopsy of the right iliac fossa mass under CT scan

Excisional biopsy done reveals an undifferentiated carcinoma, EMA^+, $KL1^+$, and NSE^+ and negative for cytokeratin 5 (CK5), ACE, calcitonin, chromogranin, synaptophysin, and protein S100 on immunohistochemistry.

2. What would you do to complete the work-up?

    a. Gastroscopy and/or colonoscopy
    b. CT scan of the neck, thorax, abdomen, and pelvis
    c. Laboratory tests and serum tumor markers
    d. Bone scan

CT scan shows in addition to cervical lymph nodes enlargement, multiple retroperitoneal and bilateral iliac adenopathies, multiple peritoneal nodules, and an 8 cm mass extending to the cul-de-sac de Douglas. No mediastinal lymph nodes or pulmonary lesions.

Laboratory tests and tumor markers were normal.

The patient received chemotherapy associating cisplatin–etoposide.

After six cycles, the disease was stable on both sides of the diaphragm.

3. What would you plan for the patient?
   a. Simple observation
   b. Radiotherapy to cervical and retroperitoneal lymph nodes
   c. Neck dissection
   d. Surgical resection of the abdominal mass and the peritoneal nodules
   e. c and d

The patient was regularly observed and examined every two months. After six months, he has no symptoms, his PS WHO score 0. His physical exam and the CT scan show no sign of disease progression. Two months later, he consults for diffuse abdominal pain, constipation, dysuria, and frequency. CT scan confirms disease progression with mainly a huge para-vesical and para-prostatic mass.

4. Which of the following management options would be appropriate at this time?
   a. Second line chemotherapy
   b. Pain killers and oral steroids
   c. Palliative radiotherapy of the pelvis
   d. Surgical resection of the paravesical mass

The patient received 45 Gy to the pelvis and was treated by oral morphine sulfate and steroids. Pain was well controlled by oral morphine, but still has constipation and urinary symptoms.

One month later, pain is no more controlled, he has loss of weight and anejaculation.

5. What would you do?
   a. Second line chemotherapy
   b. Best supportive care

We started a second line chemotherapy combining doxorubicin and ifosfamide. After two cycles, he developed hepatic metastases. He received a third line of chemotherapy (docetaxel for two cycles), but the disease kept on progressing. Specific treatment was discontinued, and the patient died two months later.

Comment

A. Plantade, P. Afchain, and C. Louvet
Hôpital Saint Antoine, Paris, France

This case describes a young man with neither past medical history nor clinical complaints. At physical exam, he presents with a cervical and supra-clavicular lymph node enlargment and a mass in the right iliac fossa.

1. First a CT scan of the neck, thorax, abdomen, and pelvis is impor-tant to complete the extension of the disease and to explore the pelvic mass. Then a surgical biopsy of a cervical lymph node has to be performed quickly to achieve a diagnosis. The surgical biopsy should be preferred to the biopsy of the right iliac fossa under CT scan. More tissue is obtained for histopathological exam and chromosomic study.

2. Histopathological exam shows an undifferentiated carcinoma on light microscopy with one positive neuroendocrine staining (NSE) on immunochemistry. Neuroendocrine feature is recog-nized only after immunochemistry is performed. Such a result con-cerns about 10% to 15% of poorly differentiated of unknown site.

   Before chemotherapy, laboratory tests and serum tumor mar-kers may be of interest (blood cells count, renal and hepatic func-tions, lactate dehydrogenase (LDH), serum chromogranin A, and serum NSE). HIV serology has to be controlled. In this type of neu-roendocrine tumors, tumor secretion of bioactive substances are rare.

   Coloscopy is not necessary because it would not change the management of the patient. Bone scan is of no interest since the patient is not complaining of bone pain.

3. Cisplatin/etoposide-based chemotherapy is recommended and is active in poorly-differentiated neuroendocrine tumors. They are chemosensitive tumors that allow complete response and some prolonged survival. Metastatic poorly-differentiated neuroendo-crine carcinomas belong to the favorable prognostic group of carcinoma of unknown primary (CUP).

   After six cycles of chemotherapy, the disease remains stable. Close observation is recommended. It can prevent the appearance of the neurototoxicity and nephrotoxicity caused by cisplatin chemotherapy. Unless the patient has local symptoms, surgery or radiotherapy is of no help since the malignant lesions are diffuse.

4. After eight months of observation, the patient is complaining of dysuria and constipation. A CT scan shows a progression, which

is mainly located in the pelvis. These symptoms are due to this pelvic progression. A second-line chemotherapy may be started. Considering the duration of tumoral stability with the cisplatin/ etoposide chemotherapy (eight months), rechallenging with the same combination can be discussed, if there is no limiting toxicity. Antalgic drugs and oral steroids should be used to improve the comfort of the patient. Pelvic radiation therapy is performed in order to control dysuria but would not treat all the metastatic sites. So its indication may be discussed. Surgery does not make sense since the pelvic infiltration is diffuse.

5. First-line chemotherapy controlled the disease during eight months. Considering the young age of the patient and the initial tumoral stability, a second-line chemotherapy has to be proposed. There is no consensus on the chemotherapy, which may be used as second-line treatment in patients with poorly differentiated neuro-endocrine carcinoma. Rechallenging with cisplatin/etoposide combination is a possibility.

Bibliography

Moertel CG, Kvols LK, O'Connell MJ, Rubin J. Treatment of neuroendocrine carcinomas with combined etoposide and cisplatin. Evidence of major therapeutic activity in the anaplastic variants of these neoplasms. Cancer 1991; 68(2):227–232.

Hainsworth JD, Greco FA. Neoplasms of unknown primary site. In: Kufe DW, Pollock RE, et al, eds. Cancer Medicine, 6th ed. Hamilton: BC Decker, Inc, 2003:2277–2290.

Fjallskog ML, Granberg DP, Welin SL, et al. Treatment with cisplatin and etoposide in patients with neuroendocrine tumors.

Mitry E, Baudin E, Ducreux M, et al. Treatment of poorly differentiated neuroendocrine tumours with etoposide and cisplatin. Cancer 2001; 92(5):1101–1107.

Greco FA, Gray J, Burris HA III, Erland JB, Morrissey LH, Hainsworth JD. Taxane-based chemotherapy for patients with carcinoma of unknown primary site. Cancer J 2001; 7(3):203–212.

A Female with Bone Metastases of an Unknown Primary Site

Roland Bugat

Institut National du Cancer (INCa), Paris, France

A 45-year-old female patient presents with thoracic and low back pain. She has no past medical history except for an excision of a benign nodule of the left breast four years ago. Her present history goes back to three months ago, she started to have low back pain mainly upon walking and running. These symptoms became permanent, accompanied by bilateral thoracic pain with mild fever. She had no respiratory, digestive, or urinary symptoms. Blood tests showed normal WBC count, no anemia, increased CRP, LDH > 6×UL, Alk ph > 2×UL.

1. Which of the following would you recommend?

    a. Chest X ray
    b. Plain films of the lumbosacral spine
    c. MRI of the lumbosacral spine
    d. Bone scan
    e. CT scan of thorax, abdomen, and pelvis
    f. Bilateral mammography

Chest X ray and lumbosacral plain films were normal. CT scan of thorax, abdomen, and pelvis showed a left renal cyst. Bone scan showed multiple hyperfixating spots over the spine and iliac bones. Bilateral mammography was normal.

2. What would be the next step?

    a. Bilateral breast MRI
    b. Bone biopsy

    c. MRI of the spine

    d. Ultrasound of the thyroid

Bone marrow biopsy showed an adenocarcinoma, CK7 positive and CK20, c-erb-B2, and hormonal receptors negative.

3. What would be your management option?

    a. FEC (fluorouracil, epirubicin, cyclophosphamide) regimen

    b. Cisplatin-based regimen

    c. Palliative bone irradiation + bisphosphonates

    d. Pain killers + bisphosphonates

    e. Best supportive care

The patient received three cycles of FEC (fluorouracil, epirubicin, cyclo-phosphamide), with no clinical improvement, she still has low back pain despite codeine analgesics. LDH and alkalin phosphatase kept on rising, and four weeks after the third cycle of FEC, she still has anemia and thrombocytopenia.

4. What would you suggest for this patient?

    a. BSC

    b. Bisphosphonates + morphine

    c. A cisplatin-based chemotherapy regimen

    d. Irradiation of the lumbo-sacral spine

We decided to treat her with the cisplatin and gemcitabine combination with pamidronate and oral morphine sulfate. Two months later she was feeling better with less low back pain but she noticed sensation loss over the chin on the left side.

    On neurological exam there was a hypoesthesia over the left side of the chin but no other cranial nerves abnormalities, neck stiffness, motor weak-ness, or babinski sign were present. MRI of the brain and the base of the skull was normal, with no intracerebral or meningeal suspicious lesion. She received two more cycles of chemotherapy, after which she had a com-plete blindness of the left eye. MRI showed fronto-parietal meningeal thick-ening with no intraparenchymal lesion. Cerebrospinal fluid contained no malignant cells.

5. What would be the most appropriate therapy you recommend to this patient?

    a. Whole brain radiation therapy

    b. Intrathecal methotrexate

    c. High dose IV methotrexate

    d. Best supportive care

The patient received one cycle of high dose methotrexate. Fifteen days later she was urgently admitted to the hospital for febrile neutropenia, severe anemia, and grade 3 thombocytopenia and then transferred to the ICU for septic shock. She stayed 72 hours in the ICU, WBC count became normal and the patient was retransferred to the ordinary unit.

6. What would you suggest in this case?
    a. Whole brain radiation therapy
    b. Intrathecal methotrexate
    c. Oral steroids
    d. High dose IV methotrexate + G-CSF support
    e. Best supportive care

Comment

A. Plantade, P. Afchain, and C. Louvet

Hôpital Saint Antoine, Paris, France

This case reports a 45-year-old woman who is complaining of thoracic and low back pain with fever. Biological exams show an increased level of CRP, LDH, and alkalin phosphatases. An infectious or a tumoral disease may be suspected.

1. A chest X ray and plain films of the lumbosacral spine are performed in order to eliminate a pleural or pulmonary disease, a costal or lumbar lesion. In case of lumbar lesion, an MRI of the spine is indicated to evaluate the neurological risk. Bilateral mammography is clearly indicated even if no clinical breast mass is palpable, first due to the clinical presentation, and second according to the previous patient's history. Then a CT scan of thorax, abdomen, and pelvis and a bone scan complete the disease extension.

2. These investigations show diffuse bone lesions that are over the spine and iliac bones and look like bone metastases. Next step is to achieve a histopathological diagnosis so a bone biopsy should be performed. In fact there is no other suspect lesion (the left renal cyst is absolutely not suspect). Waiting for the pathological results, an ultrasound of the thyroid may be performed searching for a thyroid malignancy. In case of normal mammography, a breast MRI may be helpful to rule out breast cancer. An MRI of the spine is also important to verify that the medullary canal is safe.

3. Histopathological exam shows an adenocarcinoma. The immuno-chemical staining does not help to determine the origin of the malignancy in this case. The negativity of hormonal receptors and of cerb2 does not infirm a breast origin since, at the age of 45, the majority of breast cancers have negative hormonal receptors.

Because of the high frequency of breast cancer among women and the presentation of the cancer with isolated bone metastases, it is possible to manage the patient considering she has a metastatic breast cancer. As bone metastases are already diffuse, chemotherapy should be preferred to local bone radiation therapy. Anthracycline-based chemotherapy is active in metastatic breast cancer and are still used as first-line. Biphosphonates are the current standard of care for preventing skeletal complications associated with bone metatsases (pathologic fracture, hypercalcemia of malignancy). Antalgic drugs are, of course, necessary according to the complaints of the patient.

4. After three cycles of FEC/FAC regimen, no effect has been seen. A change of strategy is needed. Cisplatin-based chemotherapy, which is usually recommended in adenocarcinoma of unknown primary (ACUP), is a possible second-line chemotherapy. Gemcitabine or paclitaxel may be added to platin compound since both are active in breast cancer and ACUP (for example, carboplatin–paclitaxel regimen or cisplatin–gemcitabine regimen). Biphosphonates should be continued in association with morphine to relieve the lumbar pain. If pain is not controlled with morphine or if a neurological risk exists, a radiation therapy of the lumbar spine should be proposed.

5. After two months of second-line chemotherapy, a new progression occurs: a meningeal carcinomatosis with neither brain localization nor malignant cells in cerebrospinal fluid. Prognosis of meningeal carcinomatosis is poor. Nevertheless a treatment could be proposed to this young patient. The goals of treatment are to improve or to stabilize the neurologic status and to prolong survival. Whole brain radiation therapy is not indicated according to the absence of cerebral localization. Intrathecal methotrexate as well as high-dose intravenous methotrexate could be proposed. Both treat the entire neuraxis. A small pharmacokinetic study suggests that high-dose intravenous methotrexate would be safer and better distributed in cerebrospinal fluid than intrathecal methotrexate.

6. After such a serious toxicity, decision to rechallenge with a chemotherapy either intrathecal or intravenous depends on the performance status of the patient. If performance status remains satisfying, a chemotherapy may be proposed. Considering the high

hematological toxicity that has taken place, intravenous methotrexate may be replaced by intrathecal methotrexate. Decreasing the dose of intravenous methotrexate is another possibility. In this case, the efficiency of intravenous methotrexate could be reduced. If performance status is impaired, best supportive care is suggested.

Bibliography

Coleman RE. Bisphosphonates in breast cancer. Ann Oncol 2005; 16(5):687–695. Epub 2005 Mar 31.

Briasoulis E, Kalofonos H, Bafaloukos D, et al. Carboplatin plus paclitaxel in unknown primary carcinoma: a phase II hellenic cooperative oncology group study. J Clin Oncol 2000; 18(17):3101–3107.

Greco FA, Burris HA III, Litchy S, et al. Gemcitabine, carboplatin, and paclitaxel for patients with carcinoma of unknown primary site: a minnie pearl cancer research network study. J Clin Oncol 2002; 20(6):1651–1656.

Fizazi K, Asselain B, Vincent-Salomon A, et al. Meningeal carcinomatosis in patients with breast cancer: clinical features, prognostic factors and results of a high-dose intrathecal methotrexate regimen. Cancer 1996; 77:1315–1323.

Yoshida S, Morii K. Intrathecal chemotherapy for patients with meningeal carcinomatosis. Oncologist 2005; 10(1):52–62.

Tetef ML, Margolin KA, Doroshow JH, et al. Pharmacokinetics and toxicity of high-dose intravenous methotrexate in the treatment of leptomeningeal carcinomatosis. Cancer Chemother Pharmacol 2000; 46(1):19–26.

Kim L, Glantz MJ. Neoplastic meningitis. Curr Treat Options Oncol 2001; 2(6): 517–527.

Index

adenocarcinoma, 81–82
  incidence, 128
  para-clinical examinations,
    128–129
  treatment, 129–130
  undifferentiated, 31
    algorithm for pathological
      diagnosis of, 28
AFP. *See* α-Fetoprotein
α-fetoprotein (AFP), 15, 40
apoptotic cell death, 170
arthroplasty, 150
asthenia, 224
axillary lymph node
  definition, 128
  dissection, 129
  metastases, 81

bcl-2, overexpression, 159, 170
β-human chorionic gonadotropin
  (β-HCG), 40
bone metastasis, 33, 44–45, 234
  isolated, 138
brain metastasis, 33
Brief Symptom Inventory (BSI), 178
bronchoalveolar carcinoma line, 163
BSI. *See* Brief Symptom Inventory

c-myc protein, 164
Cancer Diagnostic Interview Scale
  (CDIS), 181
cancer patient, psychosocial
  aspects of, 176
carcinoembryonic antigen (CEA), 18, 64
carcinoma
  differentiated, 86
  hepatocellular, 31
  small cell, 84–85
  undifferentiated, 31
    algorithm for pathological
      diagnosis of, 28
carcinoma of unknown primary site
  (CUP), 1, 12, 161
  algorithm for pathological diagnosis
    of, 27
  characteristic features of, 134
  clinical behavior of, 5–6
  clinicopathological entities of, 39
  definition, 37
  histopathological subtypes of, 38
  natural history of, 37
  prognostic predictors, 176
  QOL instruments in, 181
  treatment of, 33
  unfavorable subsets of, 43
    cervical or supraclavicular nodal
      involvement, 41

carcinoma of unknown primary site
    (CUP) (*cont.*)
  unfavorable subsets of (*cont.*)
    inguinal nodal involvement, 41
    isolated metastases, 40–41
    nodal midline distribution, 40
carcinomatosis, 79–81
  peritoneal, 44, 200
CDIS. *See* Cancer Diagnostic Interview
    Scale
cellular ploidy, 169
Center for Epidemiologic
    Studies—Depression (CES-D),
    178, 180
cerebral metastasis, 44, 141–143
cervical metastases, unknown
    primary, 51
CES-D. *See* Center for Epidemiologic
    Studies—Depression
CGH. *See* Comparative genomic
    hybridization
chemotherapy, empiric, 197
chromosome alterations, 164
cisplatin, role of, 110
cisplatin–gemcitabine regimen, 195
communication preferences, 184
comparative genomic hybridization
    (CGH), 164
cryotherapy, 149
CUP. *See* Carcinomas of unknown
    primary syndromes

depression, clinical, 177
diphosphonates, use of, 139
distress
  definition, 177
  instruments, to characterize, 178
  prevalence of, 178
  psychosocial, 177

early metastatic syndromes with
    minimal primary tumors
    (EMMP), 161
Eastern Cooperation Oncology Group
    (ECOG), 95
ECOG. *See* Eastern Cooperation
    Oncology Group

electrodes, types of, 148
empiric chemotherapy, 197
endoscopic procedures, 16–17
Epstein–Barr virus, serology for, 41
European Network of Cancer Registries
    (EUROCIM) database, 3
extragonadal germ cell
  syndrome, 40
  tumor, 82

18-F-fluorodeoxyglucose
    (FDG), 41, 135
fiberoptic bronchoscopy, 196
5-fluorouracil (5-FU), 94

gene expression profiling, 160, 166
Global Severity Index (GSI), 179
gonadal inflammation, 169
Gown's laws of immuno-histochemistry,
    30
growth factor receptors, 170

HAD-S. *See* Hospital Anxiety and
    Depression Scale
hematotoxicity, 221
hepatic resection, 137
hepatocellular carcinomas, 31
histopathological types, strategies
    for, 30–32
Hospital Anxiety and Depression Scale
    (HAD-S), 178–179
hypernephroma, 205

ICD-O. *See* International Classification
    of Diseases for Oncology
IHC. *See* Immunohistochemistry
immunohistochemistry (IHC), 134, 137
  Gown's laws of, 30
International Classification of Diseases
    for Oncology (ICD-O), 2–3

Karnofsky Performance Status, 179

lactate dehydrogenase (LDH), 62, 176
LDH. *See* Lactate dehydrogenase
liver metastasis, 33, 137
low-grade neuroendocrine carcinoma, 84
lymph nodes, 26
    cervical, 82–83
    inguinal, 84
    metastasis, 32, 135

malignant mesothelioma, 32
malignant pleural effusion, 44
malignant tumor, undifferentiated,
        30–31
matrixmetallo-proteinase (MMPs), 164
meningeal carcinomatosis, 234
mesothelioma markers, 32
metastasis, 33
    adenocarcinoma, 43
    bone, 33, 44–45, 234
    brain, 33
    cascade, 163
    cerebral, 44, 141–143
    disease, 11
    lesion, 81–82
    liver, 33, 137
    neuroendocrine carcinomas, 42
    parenchymal, 44
    phenotype, 163
    pulmonary, 33
    retroperitoneal, 202
    serous, 32
    skin, 33
    suppressor genes, 164
    syndromes, 161
microfluidics card, 160
microvessel density (MVD), 12
Minnie Pearl Cancer Research
        Network, 95
Montpellier Cancer Center, 97
morbidity, psychosocial, 179

nasopharyngeal carcinomas
        (NPC), 165
National Comprehensive Cancer
        Network (NCCN), 177

NCCN. *See* National Comprehensive
        Cancer Network
neuroendocrine carcinoma, 2, 84
    differentiated, 85–86
    malignant tumors, 42
    markers, 31
neutropenia, 219
non-Hodgkin's lymphoma, 5
nosological considerations, 160
novel therapeutic agents, 170
NPC. *See* Nasopharyngeal carcinomas

osteoblastic bone metastases, 42
osteosynthesis, 150

p53 gene, 165
palliative bone surgery, 149–150
palliative care, 187, 224
parenchymal metastases, 44
patient satisfaction, predictors
        of, 183
performance status (PS), 175
pericardiocentesis, 219
peritoneal carcinomatosis, 44, 200
    in women, 79–81
peritoneal papillary serous
        carcinomatosis, 41–42
PET. *See* Positron emission tomography
PET-FDG. *See* Positron emission
        tomography with
        18-F-fluorodeoxyglucose
physician–patient, barriers to
        information exchange, 182
physician's interpersonal skills, 180
pleural deposits, 195
poorly differentiated cancer (PDC)
        histology, 62–63
positron emission tomography (PET),
        81, 117, 128, 197
positron emission tomography with
        18-F-fluorodeoxyglucose
        (PET-FDG), 49–51
posttraumatic stress disorder, 177
prognosis, assessing, 186
prostate specific antigen (PSA), 42, 138

PSA. *See* Prostate specific antigen
psychosocial adjustment, 177
    primary factor influencing, 180
psychosocial distress, 177–179
pulmonary metastasis, 33
pulmonary nodule, solitary, 139–140

QOL. *See* Quality of life
QOL instruments in CUP, 181
quality of life (QOL) of patients, 176, 180

radiofrequency, 148–149
radiotherapy, 153
retroperitoneal metastasis, 202

SCT. *See* Spiral computed tomography
septic shock, 233
serous metastasis, 32
serum tumor markers, 18–19
skin metastasis, 33
solitary metastasis, 43
solitary pulmonary nodule, 139–140
SPIKES protocol, 184
spiral computed tomography (SCT),
    134
squamous carcinoma, 32
    cervical lymph nodes, 82–83
    chemotherapy, 122
    epidemiology, 118
    inguinal lymph nodes, 84
    radiation therapy, 121–122

SRS. *See* Stereotaxic radiosurgery
stereotactic radiotherapy, 154
stereotaxic radiosurgery (SRS), 142
surgical drainage, 219

taxanes, 170
thrombocytopenia, 219, 232
tissue lineage identification, 160
truth telling, standards for, 187
tumor cell dissemination, 164, 166
tumor mass, atypical distribution
    of, 159
tumor regression, 169

unknown primary carcinoma
    (UPC), 61
    clinical trials, 73–74
    general population of, 68
    prognostic factors, 73–74
unknown primary tumors
    (UPTs), 159
    autopsy-negative, 160
    biological aspects of, 163
    specific and nonspecific biological
        features of, 164–165
UPC. *See* Unknown primary carcinoma
UPT. *See* Unknown primary tumor

WBRT. *See* Whole-brain radiotherapy
weight loss, 224
whole-brain radiotherapy (WBRT),
    141–142

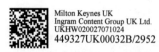

Milton Keynes UK
Ingram Content Group UK Ltd.
UKHW020027071024
449327UK00032B/2952

9 780367 453695